THE OFFICIAL U.S. GOVERNMENT MEDICARE H

MEDICARE & YOU

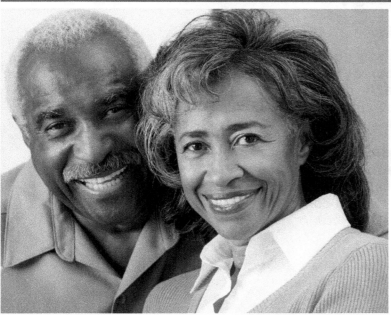
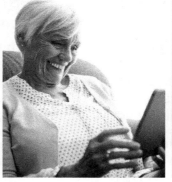
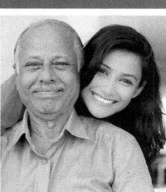
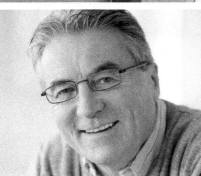
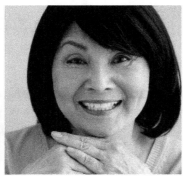
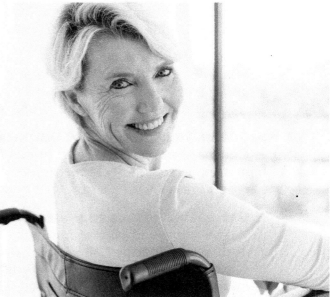

2020

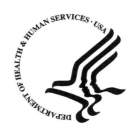
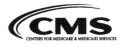

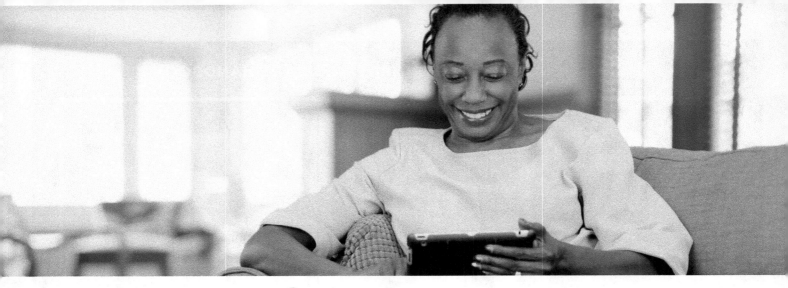

eMedicare

We're improving and modernizing the way you get Medicare information. The goal is to provide a seamless and transparent experience to help you get the information you need to make good health care choices. We're working to update the Medicare resources you already know and trust, and building new ones to work with the technology you use every day.

Get improved help with your Medicare choices
We've made it easier to find health and drug coverage that works for you. You can compare ways to get your Medicare coverage and explore how different plans work together. You can also shop and compare plans to find ones that meet your needs. Visit Medicare.gov/plan-compare.

Find out what's covered
The "What's covered" mobile app delivers reliable (Original Medicare) Part A and Part B coverage information right on your mobile device. You can download it for free on both the App Store and Google Play.

See estimated costs of outpatient procedures
Compare national average prices for certain procedures performed in both hospital outpatient departments and ambulatory surgical centers. Visit Medicare.gov/procedure-price-lookup.

Get easier access to your personal Medicare information
We've improved MyMedicare.gov to make it easier to find what you need. We added new features, like the ability to print an official copy of your Medicare card. We also connected MyMedicare.gov to Blue Button 2.0—a secure data connection that lets you share your health information with a growing number of mobile apps, third party applications, health-related services, and research programs.

Coming soon — Easily find and compare quality information
Quality information about Medicare-participating doctors, hospitals, nursing homes, dialysis facilities, and other care providers will soon be available in one easy-to-use place. Compare quality ratings, cost information, and other details to help you choose what's best for you. Coming in 2020 to Medicare.gov.

To stay on top of eMedicare improvements and other important news from Medicare, sign up to get email updates at Medicare.gov.

Contents

Get started

If you're new to Medicare:

- **Learn about your Medicare choices.** There are 2 main ways to get your Medicare coverage—Original Medicare and Medicare Advantage. See the next few pages to learn more.

- **Find out how and when you can sign up.** If you don't have Medicare Part A or Part B, see Section 1, which starts on page 15. If you don't have Medicare prescription drug coverage (Part D), see Section 6, which starts on page 73. There may be penalties if you don't sign up when you're first eligible.

- **If you have other health insurance**, see pages 20–21 to find out how it works with Medicare.

If you already have Medicare:

- **You don't need to sign up for Medicare each year.** However, you should **review your Medicare health and prescription drug coverage** and make changes if it no longer meets your needs or if you could lower your out-of-pocket expenses.

- **Mark your calendar with these important dates!** This may be the only chance you have each year to make changes to your coverage.

January 1, 2020	**New coverage begins if you made a change.** If you kept your existing coverage and your plan's costs or benefits changed, those changes will also start on this date.
January 1 to March 31, 2020	**If you're in a Medicare Advantage Plan**, you can make a change to a different Medicare Advantage Plan or switch back to Original Medicare (and join a stand-alone Medicare Prescription Drug Plan) once during this time. Any changes you make will be effective the first of the month after the plan gets your request. See page 65.
October 1, 2020	**Start comparing your current coverage with other options.** You may be able to save money. Visit Medicare.gov/plan-compare.
October 15 to December 7, 2020	**Change your Medicare health or prescription drug coverage for 2021, if you decide to.** This includes returning to Original Medicare or joining a Medicare Advantage Plan.

✪ Pages 5–9 provide an overview of your Medicare options.

What are the parts of Medicare?

Part A (Hospital Insurance)

Helps cover:

- Inpatient care in hospitals
- Skilled nursing facility care
- Hospice care
- Home health care

See pages 25–28.

Part B (Medical Insurance)

Helps cover:

- Services from doctors and other health care providers
- Outpatient care
- Home health care
- Durable medical equipment (like wheelchairs, walkers, hospital beds, and other equipment)
- Many preventive services (like screenings, shots or vaccines, and yearly "Wellness" visits)

See pages 29–49.

Part D (Prescription drug coverage)

Helps cover:

- Cost of prescription drugs (including many recommended shots or vaccines)

Part D plans are run by private insurance companies that follow rules set by Medicare.

See pages 73–82.

Your Medicare options

When you first enroll in Medicare and during certain times of the year, you can choose how you get your Medicare coverage. There are 2 main ways to get Medicare:

Original Medicare

- Original Medicare includes Medicare Part A (Hospital Insurance) and Part B (Medical Insurance).
- If you want drug coverage, you can join a separate Part D plan.
- To help pay your out-of-pocket costs in Original Medicare (like your 20% coinsurance), you can also shop for and buy supplemental coverage.
- Can use any doctor or hospital that takes Medicare, anywhere in the U.S.

☑ **Part A**

☑ **Part B**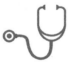

You can add:

☐ **Part D**

You can also add:

☐ **Supplemental coverage**

(Some examples include coverage from a Medicare Supplement Insurance (Medigap) policy, or coverage from a former employer or union.)

See Section 3, which starts on page 51 to learn more about Original Medicare.

Medicare Advantage
(also known as Part C)

- Medicare Advantage is an "all in one" alternative to Original Medicare. These "bundled" plans include Part A, Part B, and usually Part D.
- Plans may have lower out-of-pocket costs than Original Medicare.
- In most cases, you'll need to use doctors who are in the plan's network.
- Most plans offer extra benefits that Original Medicare doesn't cover— like vision, hearing, dental, and more.

☑ **Part A**

☑ **Part B**

Most plans include:

☑ **Part D**

☑ **Extra benefits**

Some plans also include:

☐ **Lower out-of-pocket costs**

See Section 4, which starts on page 55, to learn more about Medicare Advantage.

AT A GLANCE

Original Medicare vs. Medicare Advantage

 ## Doctor and hospital choice

Original Medicare	Medicare Advantage
You can go to **any doctor or hospital that takes Medicare, anywhere in the U.S.**	In most cases, you'll need to use **doctors who are in the plan's network** (for non-emergency or non-urgent care). Ask your doctor if they participate in any Medicare Advantage Plans.
In most cases, you **don't need** a referral to see a specialist.	You **may need** to get a referral to see a specialist.

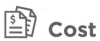 ## Cost

Original Medicare	Medicare Advantage
For Part B-covered services, **you usually pay 20% of the Medicare-approved amount** after you meet your deductible.	**Out-of-pocket costs vary**—plans may have lower out-of-pocket costs for certain services.
You **pay a premium (monthly payment) for Part B**. If you choose to buy prescription drug coverage (Part D), you'll pay that premium separately.	You may **pay a premium for the plan** in addition to a monthly **premium for Part B**. (Most include prescription drug coverage.) Plans may have a $0 premium or may help pay all or part of your Part B premiums.
There's **no yearly limit** on what you pay out-of-pocket, unless you have supplemental coverage (like a Medigap policy).	Plans have a **yearly limit** on what you pay out-of-pocket for Medicare Part A- and B-covered services. Once you reach your plan's limit, you'll pay nothing for Part A- and Part B-covered services for the rest of the year.
You **can get** supplemental coverage (like a Medigap policy) to help pay your remaining out-of-pocket costs (like your 20% coinsurance). Or, you can use coverage from a former employer or union, or Medicaid.	You **can't buy or use** separate supplemental coverage.

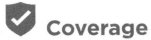 Coverage

Original Medicare	Medicare Advantage
Original Medicare covers most medically necessary services and supplies in hospitals, doctors' offices, and other health care settings.	Plans must cover all of the medically necessary services that Original Medicare covers. Most plans **may offer extra benefits that Original Medicare doesn't cover**—like vision, hearing, dental, and more. Plans can now cover more of these benefits than they have in the past. See page 56.
You can join a **separate Medicare Prescription Drug Plan (Part D)** to get drug coverage.	**Prescription drug coverage is included** in most plans.
In most cases, you don't have to get a service or supply approved ahead of time for it to be covered.	In some cases, you have to get a service or supply approved ahead of time for it to be covered by the plan.

✈ Travel

Original Medicare	Medicare Advantage
Original Medicare generally **doesn't cover care outside the U.S.** You may be able to buy a Medigap policy that covers care outside the U.S.	Plans generally **don't cover care outside the U.S.** Also, plans usually don't cover non-emergency care you get outside of your plan's network.

These topics are explained in more detail throughout this book.
- **Original Medicare:** See Section 3 (starting on page 51).
- **Medicare Advantage:** See Section 4 (starting on page 55).
- **Prescription drug coverage (Part D):** See Section 6 (starting on page 73).

Look for 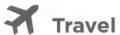 throughout this book to see comparisons between Original Medicare and Medicare Advantage.

Get the most out of Medicare

Get help choosing the coverage option that's right for you:

- Get free, personalized counseling from your State Health Insurance Assistance Program (SHIP)—see pages 109–112 for the phone number.
- Call 1-800-MEDICARE (1-800-633-4227). TTY users can call 1-877-486-2048.
- Visit the Medicare Plan Finder at Medicare.gov/plan-compare.

Get the most value out of your health care

We want to make sure you have the information you need to make the best decisions about your health care. This includes giving you access to cost and quality information up front, so you can compare and choose the providers and services that give you the most value. Look for 🔍 throughout this book to learn about the different ways to shop for your health care.

Get free help with your Medicare questions

For general Medicare questions, visit Medicare.gov, or call 1-800-MEDICARE. See pages 101–108 to learn about other resources.

Get preventive services

Ask your doctor or other health care provider which preventive services (like screenings, shots or vaccines, and yearly "Wellness" visits) you need to get. Medicare covers many common preventive services at no cost to you. See pages 30–49 and look for the 🍎 to learn more.

Get help paying for health care

Find out if you can get help paying your health and prescription drug costs. Go to Section 7, which starts on page 83, to see if you may qualify.

Go paperless

Help save tax dollars and paper by switching to the electronic version of this handbook. You'll stop getting a paper copy each fall. Visit Medicare.gov/gopaperless, or log into your MyMedicare.gov account to switch to the electronic handbook. See page 101 for details.

Index of topics

⭐ **Note:** The page numbers shown in **bold** provide the most detailed information.

⭐ **Note:** The page numbers shown in **bold** provide the most detailed information.

⭐ **Note:** The page numbers shown in **bold** provide the most detailed information.

⭐ **Note:** The page numbers shown in **bold** provide the most detailed information.

⭐ **Note:** The page numbers shown in **bold** provide the most detailed information.

SECTION 1

Signing up for Medicare

Some people get Part A and Part B automatically

If you're already getting benefits from Social Security or the Railroad Retirement Board (RRB), you'll automatically get Part A and Part B starting the first day of the month you turn 65. (If your birthday is on the first day of the month, Part A and Part B will start the first day of the prior month.)

If you're under 65 and have a disability, you'll automatically get Part A and Part B after you get disability benefits from Social Security or certain disability benefits from the RRB for 24 months.

> If you live in Puerto Rico, you don't automatically get Part B. You must sign up for it. See page 16 for more information.

If you have ALS (amyotrophic lateral sclerosis, also called Lou Gehrig's disease), you'll get Part A and Part B automatically the month your Social Security disability benefits begin.

If you're automatically enrolled, you'll get your red, white, and blue Medicare card in the mail 3 months before your 65th birthday or 25th month of disability benefits. If you do nothing, you'll keep Part B and will have to pay Part B premiums through your Social Security benefits. You can choose not to keep Part B, but if you decide you want Part B later, you may have to wait to enroll and pay a penalty for as long as you have Part B. See page 22.

Note: If you need to replace your card because it's damaged or lost, sign in to your MyMedicare.gov account to print an official copy of your Medicare card. If you don't have an account, visit MyMedicare.gov to create one. If you need to replace your card because you think that someone else is using your number, call us at 1-800-MEDICARE (1-800-633-4227). TTY users can call 1-877-486-2048.

⭐ **Note:** Definitions of blue words are on pages 113–116.

Some people have to sign up for Part A and/or Part B

If you're close to 65, but not getting Social Security or Railroad Retirement Board (RRB) benefits, you'll need to sign up for Medicare. Contact Social Security 3 months before you turn 65. You can also apply for Part A and Part B at ssa.gov/benefits/medicare. If you worked for a railroad, contact the RRB. **In most cases, if you don't sign up for Part B when you're first eligible, you may have a delay in getting Medicare coverage in the future (in some cases over a year), and you may have to pay a late enrollment penalty for as long as you have Part B. See page 22.**

If you have End-Stage Renal Disease (ESRD) and you want Medicare, you'll need to sign up. Contact Social Security to find out when and how to sign up for Part A and Part B. For more information, visit Medicare.gov/publications to view the booklet "Medicare Coverage of Kidney Dialysis & Kidney Transplant Services."

Important! **If you live in Puerto Rico and get benefits from Social Security or the RRB,** you'll automatically get Part A the first day of the month you turn 65 or after you get disability benefits for 24 months. **However, if you want Part B, you'll need to sign up for it by completing an "Application for Enrollment in Part B Form" (CMS-40B). If you don't sign up for Part B when you're first eligible, you may have to pay a late enrollment penalty for as long as you have Part B. See page 22.** Visit CMS.gov/medicare/cms-forms/cms-forms/cms-forms-items/cms017339.html to get Form CMS-40B in English or Spanish. Contact your local Social Security office or RRB for more information.

Where can I get more information?
Call Social Security at 1-800-772-1213 for more information about your Medicare eligibility and to sign up for Part A and/or Part B. TTY users can call 1-800-325-0778. If you worked for a railroad or get RRB benefits, call the RRB at 1-877-772-5772. TTY users can call 1-312-751-4701.

You can also get free, personalized health insurance counseling from your State Health Insurance Assistance Program (SHIP). See pages 109–112 for the phone number.

> After you've enrolled in Medicare, you'll need to decide how to get your Medicare coverage. See pages 5–9 for more information.

If I'm not automatically enrolled, when can I sign up?

If you're not automatically enrolled in premium-free Part A, you can sign up for Part A once your Initial Enrollment Period starts. Your Part A coverage will start 6 months before the month you apply for Medicare (or Social Security/RRB benefits), but no earlier than the first month you turn 65. However, you can only sign up for Part B (or Part A if you have to buy it) during the times listed below.

Important! **Remember, in most cases, if you don't sign up for Part A (if you have to buy it) and Part B when you're first eligible, you may have to pay a late enrollment penalty. See page 22.**

Initial Enrollment Period

You can first sign up for Part A and/or Part B during the 7-month period that begins 3 months before the month you turn 65, includes the month you turn 65, and ends 3 months after the month you turn 65.

If you sign up for Part A and/or Part B during the first 3 months of your Initial Enrollment Period, in most cases, your coverage starts the first day of your birthday month. However, if your birthday is on the first day of the month, your coverage will start the first day of the prior month.

If you enroll in Part A (that you have to pay for) and/or Part B the month you turn 65 or during the last 3 months of your Initial Enrollment Period, the start date for your Part B coverage will be delayed.

Special Enrollment Period

After your Initial Enrollment Period is over, you may have a chance to sign up for Medicare during a Special Enrollment Period. If you didn't sign up for Part B (or Part A if you have to buy it) when you were first eligible because you're covered under a group health plan based on current employment (your own, a spouse's, or a family member's (if you have a disability)), you can sign up for Part A and/or Part B:

- Anytime you're still covered by the group health plan
- During the 8-month period that begins the month after the employment ends or the coverage ends, whichever happens first

Usually, you don't pay a late enrollment penalty if you sign up during a Special Enrollment Period. This Special Enrollment Period doesn't apply to people who are eligible for Medicare based on End-Stage Renal Disease (ESRD). It also doesn't apply if you're still in your Initial Enrollment Period.

Note: If you have a disability, and the group health plan coverage is based on the current employment of a family member (other than a spouse), the employer offering the group health plan must have 100 or more employees for you to get a Special Enrollment Period.

Important!   **COBRA (Consolidated Omnibus Budget Reconciliation Act) coverage, retiree health plans, VA coverage, and individual health coverage (like through the Health Insurance Marketplace) aren't considered coverage based on current employment.** You aren't eligible for a Special Enrollment Period to sign up for Medicare when that coverage ends. To avoid paying a higher premium, make sure you sign up for Medicare when you're first eligible. See page 81 for more information about COBRA coverage.

To learn more about enrollment periods, visit Medicare.gov, or call 1-800-MEDICARE (1-800-633-4227). TTY users can call 1-877-486-2048.

General Enrollment Period

If you didn't sign up for Part A (if you have to buy it) and/or Part B (for which you must pay premiums) during your Initial Enrollment Period, and you don't qualify for a Special Enrollment Period, you can sign up between January 1–March 31 each year. **Your coverage won't start until July 1 of that year, and you may have to pay a higher Part A and/or Part B premium for late enrollment.** See pages 21–22.

Should I get Part B?

This information can help you decide if you should get Part B.

Employer or union coverage: If you or your spouse (or family member if you have a disability) **is still working** and you have health coverage through that employer or union, contact your employer or union benefits administrator to find out how your coverage works with Medicare. This includes federal or state employment and active-duty military service. It might be to your advantage to delay Part B enrollment.

Note: Remember, coverage based on current employment doesn't include:
- COBRA
- Retiree coverage
- VA coverage
- Individual health coverage (like through the Health Insurance Marketplace)

TRICARE: If you have TRICARE (health care program for active-duty and retired service members and their families), **you generally must enroll in Part A and Part B when you're first eligible to keep your TRICARE coverage.** However, if you're an active-duty service member or an active-duty family member, you don't have to enroll in Part B to keep your TRICARE coverage. For more information, contact TRICARE. See page 82.

> If you have CHAMPVA coverage, you must enroll in Part A and Part B to keep it. Call 1-800-733-8387 for more information about CHAMPVA.

Medicaid: If you have Medicaid, you should sign up for Part B. Medicare will pay first, and Medicaid will pay second. Medicaid may be able to help pay your Medicare out-of-pocket costs (like premiums, deductibles, coinsurances, and copayments).

Health Insurance Marketplace: Even if you have Marketplace coverage, you should enroll in Medicare when you're first eligible to avoid the risk of a delay in Medicare coverage and the possibility of a Medicare late enrollment penalty. It's important to terminate (end) your Marketplace coverage in a timely manner to avoid an overlap in coverage. Once you're considered eligible for or enrolled in Part A, you won't qualify for help through the Marketplace for paying your Marketplace plan premiums or other medical costs. If you continue to get help paying your Marketplace plan premium after you have Medicare, you may have to pay back the help you got when you file your taxes. Visit **HealthCare.gov** to connect to the Marketplace in your state and learn more. You can also find out how to end your Marketplace plan or Marketplace financial help when your Medicare enrollment begins. You can also call the Marketplace Call Center at 1-800-318-2596. TTY users can call 1-855-889-4325.

Health savings accounts (HSAs): You can't contribute to your HSA once your Medicare coverage begins. However, you may use money that's already in your HSA after you enroll in Medicare to help pay for deductibles, premiums (if you're billed directly), copayments, or coinsurance. If you or your employer contribute to your HSA after your Medicare coverage starts, you may have to pay a tax penalty. If you'd like to continue contributing to your employer-sponsored HSA without penalty after you turn 65, you shouldn't apply for Medicare, Social Security, or Railroad Retirement Board (RRB) benefits.

Remember, premium-free Part A coverage begins 6 months before the month you apply for Medicare (or Social Security/RRB benefits), but no earlier than the month you turn 65. To avoid a tax penalty, you should stop contributing to your HSA at least 6 months before you apply for Medicare.

A Medicare Advantage Medical Savings Account (MSA) Plan might be an option if you'd like to continue to get health benefits through an HSA-like structure. See page 55 for more information.

How does my other insurance work with Medicare?

When you have other insurance and Medicare, there are rules for whether Medicare or your other insurance pays first.

If you have **retiree** insurance (insurance from your or your spouse's former employment)...	Medicare pays first.
If you're 65 or older, have group health plan coverage based on your or your spouse's **current** employment, and the employer has **20 or more employees**...	Your group health plan pays first.
If you're 65 or older, have group health plan coverage based on your or your spouse's **current** employment, and the employer has **fewer than 20 employees**...	Medicare pays first.
If you're under 65 and have a disability, have group health plan coverage based on your or a family member's **current** employment, and the employer has **100 or more employees**...	Your group health plan pays first.
If you're under 65 and have a disability, have group health plan coverage based on your or a family member's **current** employment, and the employer has **fewer than 100 employees**...	Medicare pays first.
If you have Medicare because of End-Stage Renal Disease (ESRD)...	Your group health plan will pay first for the first 30 months after you become eligible to enroll in Medicare. Medicare will pay first after this 30-month period.
If you have Medicaid...	Medicare pays first.

Here are some important facts to remember about how other insurance works with Medicare covered services:

- The insurance that pays first (primary payer) pays up to the limits of its coverage.
- The insurance that pays second (secondary payer) only pays if there are costs the primary insurer didn't cover.
- The secondary payer (which may be Medicare) might not pay all of the uncovered costs.
- If your employer insurance is the secondary payer, you might need to enroll in Part B before your insurance will pay.

For more information, visit Medicare.gov/publications to view the booklet "Medicare & Other Health Benefits: Your Guide to Who Pays First." You can also call 1-800-MEDICARE (1-800-633-4227) for more information. TTY users can call 1-877-486-2048.

If you have other insurance or changes to your insurance, you need to let Medicare know by calling Medicare's Benefits Coordination & Recovery Center (BCRC) at 1-855-798-2627. TTY users can call 1-855-797-2627.

Important! If you have Part A, you may get a Health Coverage form (IRS Form 1095-B) from Medicare by early 2020. This form verifies that you had health coverage in 2019. Keep the form for your records. Not everyone will get this form. If you don't get Form 1095-B, don't worry, you don't need to have it to file your taxes.

How much does Part A coverage cost?

You usually don't pay a monthly premium for Part A coverage if you or your spouse paid Medicare taxes while working for a certain amount of time. This is sometimes called premium-free Part A. If you aren't eligible for premium-free Part A, you may be able to buy Part A.

In most cases, if you choose to **buy** Part A, you must also have Part B and pay monthly premiums for both. If you choose NOT to buy Part A, you can still buy Part B.

People who have to buy Part A will pay up to $458 each month in 2020.

The **2020** Part A premium amounts weren't available at the time of printing. To get the most up-to-date cost information, visit Medicare.gov later this fall.

What's the Part A late enrollment penalty?
If you aren't eligible for premium-free Part A, and you don't buy it when you're first eligible, your monthly premium may go up 10%. You'll have to pay the higher premium for twice the number of years you could've had Part A but didn't sign up.

Example: If you were eligible for Part A for 2 years but didn't sign up, you'll have to pay a 10% higher premium for 4 years.

How much does Part B coverage cost?

The standard Part B premium amount in 2020 is $144.60. Most people pay the standard Part B premium amount.

If your modified adjusted gross income as reported on your IRS tax return from 2 years ago is above a certain amount, you'll pay the standard premium amount and an Income Related Monthly Adjustment Amount, also known as IRMAA. IRMAA is an extra charge added to your premium. Visit **Medicare.gov/your-medicare-costs/part-b-costs**, or call 1-800-MEDICARE (1-800-633-4227) for more information. TTY users can call 1-877-486-2048.

Note: You'll also pay an extra amount for your Part D premium (if applicable). See page 76.

If you have to pay an extra amount and you disagree (for example, you have a life event that lowers your income), visit **socialsecurity.gov** or call Social Security at 1-800-772-1213. TTY users can call 1-800-325-0778.

What's the Part B late enrollment penalty?

Important! **If you don't sign up for Part B when you're first eligible, you may have to pay a late enrollment penalty for as long as you have Part B.** Your monthly premium for Part B may go up 10% for each full 12 months in the period that you could've had Part B, but didn't sign up for it. If you're allowed to sign up for Part B during a Special Enrollment Period, you usually don't pay a late enrollment penalty. See page 17.

> **Example:** Mr. Smith's Initial Enrollment Period ended December 2016. He waited to sign up for Part B until March 2019 during the General Enrollment Period. His coverage starts July 1, 2019. His Part B premium penalty is 20%, and he'll have to pay this penalty for as long as he has Part B. (Even though Mr. Smith wasn't covered a total of 27 months, this included only 2 full 12-month periods.)

To learn how to get help with Medicare costs, see Section 7, which starts on page 83.

How can I pay my Part B premium?

If you get Social Security or Railroad Retirement Board (RRB) benefits, your Medicare Part B (Medical Insurance) premium will be deducted from your benefit payment.

If you're a federal retiree with an annuity from OPM and not entitled to RRB or SSA benefits, you may request to have your Part B premiums deducted from your annuity. Call 1-800-MEDICARE (1-800-633-4227) to make your request. TTY users can call 1-877-486-2048.

If you don't get these benefit payments, you'll get a bill. If you choose to buy Medicare Part A (Hospital Insurance), you'll always get a bill for your premium. There are 4 ways to pay these bills:

1. **Pay by check or money order.** Write your Medicare Number on your payment, and mail it with your payment coupon to:

   Medicare Premium Collection Center
   P.O. Box 790355
   St. Louis, MO 63179-0355

2. **Pay by credit/debit card.** To do this, complete the bottom portion of the payment coupon on your Medicare Premium Bill, and mail it to the address above. Payments submitted without the bottom portion of the payment coupon may not be processed.

3. **Sign up for Medicare Easy Pay.** This is a free service that automatically deducts your premium payments from your savings or checking account each month. Visit Medicare.gov and search for "Easy Pay," or call 1-800-MEDICARE to find out how to sign up.

4. **Use your financial institution's Online Bill Payment service.** Electronic online bill payments are a secure and fast way to make your payment from a checking or savings account. Ask your financial institution if it allows customers to pay bills online. Not all financial institutions offer this service and some may charge a fee. You'll need to give your financial institution this information:

   - **Account number:** This is your Medicare Number. It's important that you use the exact number on your red, white, and blue Medicare card, but without the dashes.
   - **Biller name:** CMS Medicare Insurance
   - **Remittance address:**
     Medicare Premium Collection Center
     P.O. Box 790355
     St. Louis, MO 63179-0355

Note to RRB Annuitants: If you get a bill from the RRB, mail your premium payments to:

   RRB Medicare Premium Payments
   P.O. Box 979024
   St. Louis, MO 63197-9000

If you have questions about your premiums, call 1-800-MEDICARE (1-800-633-4227). TTY users can call 1-877-486-2048. If you need to change your address on your bill, call Social Security at 1-800-772-1213. TTY users can call 1-800-325-0778. If your bills are from the RRB, call 1-877-772-5772. TTY users can call 1-312-751-4701.

If you'd like more information about paying your Medicare premiums, visit Medicare.gov to view the brochure "Understanding the Medicare Premium Bill Form (CMS-500)."

Important! If you need help paying your Part B premium, see pages 86–88.

SECTION 2

Find out if Medicare covers your test, service, or item

What services does Medicare cover?

Medicare Part A and Part B cover certain medical services and supplies in hospitals, doctors' offices, and other health care settings. Prescription drug coverage is provided through Medicare Part D.

If you have both Part A and Part B, you can get all of the Medicare-covered services listed in this section, whether you have Original Medicare or a Medicare Advantage Plan or other Medicare health plan.

What does Part A cover?

Part A (Hospital Insurance) helps cover:

- Inpatient care in a hospital
- Inpatient care in a skilled nursing facility **(not custodial or long-term care)**
- Hospice care
- Home health care
- Inpatient care in a religious nonmedical health care institution

You can find out if you have Part A by looking at your red, white, and blue Medicare card. If you have it, it will be listed as "HOSPITAL" and will have an effective date. If you have Original Medicare, you'll use this card to get your Medicare-covered services. If you join a Medicare Advantage Plan or Medicare health plan, in most cases, you must use the card from the plan to get your Medicare-covered services.

You can get Original Medicare Part A coverage information right on your mobile device. Download the "What's covered" mobile app for free on the App Store or Google Play.

⭐ **Note:** Definitions of blue words are on pages 113–116.

What do I pay for Part A-covered services?

Copayments, coinsurance, or deductibles may apply for each service listed on the following pages.

If you're in a Medicare Advantage Plan or have other insurance (like a Medigap policy, Medicaid, or employer or union coverage), your copayments, coinsurance, or deductibles may be different. Contact the plans you're interested in to find out about the costs, or visit the Medicare Plan Finder at Medicare.gov/plan-compare. Or, call 1-800-MEDICARE (1-800-633-4227). TTY users can call 1-877-486-2048.

Part A-covered services

Blood

If the hospital gets blood from a blood bank at no charge, you won't have to pay for it or replace it. If the hospital has to buy blood for you, you must either pay the hospital costs for the first 3 units of blood you get in a calendar year or have the blood donated by you or someone else.

Home health services

Home health benefits are covered under Part A and/or Part B. See page 40 for more information about home health services.

Hospice care

To qualify for hospice care, a hospice doctor and your doctor (if you have one) must certify that you're terminally ill, meaning you have a life expectancy of 6 months or less. When you agree to hospice care, you're agreeing to palliative care (comfort care) rather than care to cure your illness. You also must sign a statement choosing hospice care instead of other Medicare-covered treatments for your terminal illness and related conditions. Coverage includes:

- All items and services needed for pain relief and symptom management
- Medical, nursing, and social services
- Drugs
- Durable medical equipment
- Aide and homemaker services
- Other covered services, as well as services Medicare usually doesn't cover, like spiritual and grief counseling

A Medicare-certified hospice usually gives hospice care in your home or other facility where you live, like a nursing home or an assisted nursing facility.

Hospice care doesn't pay for your stay in a facility (room and board) unless the hospice medical team determines that you need short-term inpatient stays for pain and symptom management that can't be addressed at home. These stays must be in a Medicare-approved facility, like a hospice facility, hospital, or skilled nursing facility that contracts with the hospice. Medicare also covers inpatient respite care, which is care you get in a Medicare-approved facility so that your usual caregiver (family member or friend) can rest. You can stay up to 5 days each time you get respite care. Medicare will pay for covered services for health problems that aren't related to your terminal illness or related conditions. After 6 months, you can continue to get hospice care as long as the hospice medical director or hospice doctor recertifies (at a face-to-face meeting) that you're terminally ill.

- You pay nothing for hospice care.
- You pay a copayment of up to $5 per prescription for outpatient prescription drugs for pain and symptom management.
- You pay 5% of the Medicare-approved amount for inpatient respite care.

> Original Medicare will be billed for your hospice care, even if you're in a Medicare Advantage Plan.

Hospital care (inpatient care)

Medicare covers semi-private rooms, meals, general nursing, and drugs as part of your inpatient treatment, and other hospital services and supplies. This includes care you get in acute care hospitals, critical access hospitals, inpatient rehabilitation facilities, long-term care hospitals, inpatient care as part of a qualifying clinical research study, and inpatient mental health care given in a psychiatric hospital or psychiatric unit within a hospital. This doesn't include private-duty nursing, a television or phone in your room (if there's a separate charge for these items), or personal care items, like razors or slipper socks. It also doesn't include a private room, unless medically necessary. If you have Part B, it generally covers 80% of the Medicare-approved amount for doctor's services you get while you're in a hospital.

- You pay a deductible of $1,408 and no coinsurance for days 1–60 of each benefit period.
- You pay a coinsurance amount of $352 per day for days 61–90 of each benefit period.
- You pay a coinsurance amount per "lifetime reserve day" after day 90 of each benefit period (up to 60 days over your lifetime).
- You pay all costs for each day after you use all the lifetime reserve days.
- Inpatient psychiatric care in a freestanding psychiatric hospital is limited to 190 days in a lifetime.

Am I an inpatient or outpatient?

Staying overnight in a hospital doesn't always mean you're an inpatient. Your doctor must order your hospital admission and the hospital must formally admit you for you to be an inpatient. Without the formal inpatient admission, you're still an outpatient, even if you stay overnight in a regular hospital bed, and/or you're getting emergency department services, observation services, outpatient surgery, lab tests, or X-rays. **You or your caregiver should always ask the hospital and/or your doctor if you're an inpatient or an outpatient each day during your stay, since it affects what you pay and can affect whether you'll qualify for Part A coverage in a skilled nursing facility. You can also ask a hospital social worker or patient advocate if you're unsure.**

A "Medicare Outpatient Observation Notice" (MOON) is a document that lets you know you're an outpatient (and not an inpatient) in a hospital or critical access hospital. You must receive this notice if you're getting observation services as an outpatient for more than 24 hours. The MOON will tell you why you're an outpatient receiving observation services, rather than an inpatient. It will also let you know how this may affect what you pay while in the hospital, and for care you get after leaving the hospital.

Religious non-medical health care institution (inpatient care)

In these facilities, religious beliefs don't allow for medical care. If you qualify for hospital or skilled nursing facility care, Medicare will only cover the inpatient, non-religious, non-medical items and services. Examples are room and board, or any items and services that don't require a doctor's order or prescription, like unmedicated wound dressings or use of a simple walker.

Skilled nursing facility care

Medicare covers semi-private rooms, meals, skilled nursing and rehabilitative services, and other medically necessary services and supplies furnished in a skilled nursing facility. These services are only covered after a 3-day minimum, medically necessary, inpatient hospital stay for a related illness or injury. You may get coverage of skilled nursing care or skilled therapy care if it's necessary to improve or maintain your current condition. If the skilled nursing facility decides you should be discharged based solely on a lack of improvement, and not because you no longer require skilled nursing or therapy care, you can appeal this decision. See page 92 for your rights when you think you're being discharged too soon.

To qualify for skilled nursing facility care coverage, your doctor must certify that you need daily skilled care (like intravenous fluids/medications or physical therapy) which, as a practical matter, can only be provided to you as an inpatient of a skilled nursing facility. Medicare doesn't cover long-term care (see page 50) or custodial care.

You pay:
- Nothing for the first 20 days of each benefit period
- A coinsurance amount of $176 per day for days 21–100 of each benefit period
- All costs for each day after day 100 in a benefit period

> If your doctor is participating in an Accountable Care Organization (or other type of Medicare initiative) that's approved for a Skilled Nursing Facility 3-Day Rule Waiver, you may not need to have a 3-day inpatient hospital stay before getting skilled nursing facility care coverage. See page 106.

What does Part B cover?

Medicare Part B (Medical Insurance) helps cover medically necessary doctors' services, outpatient care, home health services, durable medical equipment, mental health services, and other medical services. Part B also covers many preventive services. You can find out if you have Part B by looking at your red, white, and blue Medicare card. If you have it, it will be listed as "MEDICAL" and will have an effective date. See pages 30–49 for a list of common Part B-covered services and general descriptions. Medicare may cover some services and tests more often than the timeframes listed if needed to diagnose or treat a condition. To find out if Medicare covers a service not on this list, visit **Medicare.gov/coverage**, or call 1-800-MEDICARE (1-800-633-4227). TTY users can call 1-877-486-2048.

> You can get Original Medicare Part B coverage information right on your mobile device. Download the "What's covered" mobile app for free on the App Store or Google Play.

What do I pay for Part B-covered services?

The alphabetical list on the following pages gives general information about what you pay if you have Original Medicare and see doctors or other health care providers who accept assignment. See page 53. You'll pay more if you see doctors or providers who don't accept assignment. **If you're in a Medicare Advantage Plan or have other insurance (like a Medigap policy, Medicaid, or employer or union coverage), your copayments, coinsurance, or deductibles may be different.**

Under Original Medicare, if the Part B deductible ($198 in 2020) applies, you must pay all costs (up to the Medicare-approved amount) until you meet the yearly Part B deductible. Visit **Medicare.gov** later this fall to find out how much the 2020 Part B deductible will be. After your deductible is met, Medicare begins to pay its share and you typically pay 20% of the Medicare-approved amount of the service, if the doctor or other health care provider accepts assignment. **There's no yearly limit for what you pay out-of-pocket.**

You pay nothing for most covered preventive services if you get the services from a doctor or other qualified health care provider who accepts assignment. However, for some preventive services, you may have to pay a deductible, coinsurance, or both. These costs may also apply if you get a preventive service in the same visit as a non-preventive service.

> Medicare Advantage Plans have a yearly limit on your out-of-pocket costs for medical services. See page 59 to learn more and to find out what affects your Medicare Advantage Plan costs.

Part B-covered services

> You'll see this apple next to the preventive services on pages 30-49.

Abdominal aortic aneurysm screening

Medicare covers a one-time abdominal aortic aneurysm screening ultrasound for people at risk. You must get a referral from your doctor or other qualified health care provider. You pay nothing for the screening if the doctor or other qualified health care practitioner accepts assignment.

Note: If you have a family history of abdominal aortic aneurysms, or you're a man 65–75 and you've smoked at least 100 cigarettes in your lifetime, you're considered at risk.

Advance care planning

Medicare covers voluntary advance care planning as part of the yearly "Wellness" visit. This is planning for care you would want to get if you become unable to speak for yourself. You can talk about an advance directive with your health care professional, and he or she can help you fill out the forms, if you want to. An advance directive is an important legal document that records your wishes about medical treatment at a future time, if you're not able to make decisions about your care. You can update your advance directives at any time. You pay nothing if it's provided as part of the yearly "Wellness" visit and the doctor or other qualified health care provider accepts assignment.

Note: Medicare may also cover this service as part of your medical treatment. When advance care planning isn't part of your yearly "Wellness" visit, the Part B deductible and coinsurance apply.

> Visit the Eldercare Locator at **eldercare.acl.gov** to find help in your community with advance directives.

Alcohol misuse screening and counseling

Medicare covers one alcohol misuse screening per year for adults with Medicare (including pregnant women) who use alcohol, but don't meet the medical criteria for alcohol dependency. If your health care provider determines you're misusing alcohol, you can get up to 4 brief face-to-face counseling sessions per year (if you're competent and alert during counseling). You must get counseling in a primary care setting (like a doctor's office). You pay nothing if the doctor or other qualified health care provider accepts assignment.

Ambulance services

Medicare covers ground ambulance transportation when you need to be transported to a hospital, critical access hospital, or skilled nursing facility for medically necessary services, and transportation in any other vehicle could endanger your health. Medicare may pay for emergency ambulance transportation in an airplane or helicopter to a hospital if you need immediate and rapid ambulance transportation that ground transportation can't provide.

In some cases, Medicare may pay for limited, medically necessary, non-emergency ambulance transportation if you have a written order from your doctor stating that ambulance transportation is medically necessary. An example may be a medically necessary ambulance transport to a dialysis facility for someone with End-Stage Renal Disease (ESRD).

Medicare will only cover ambulance services to the nearest appropriate medical facility that's able to give you the care you need.

You pay 20% of the Medicare-approved amount, and the Part B deductible applies.

Ambulatory surgical centers

Medicare covers the facility service fees related to approved surgical procedures provided in an ambulatory surgical center (facility where surgical procedures are performed, and the patient is expected to be released within 24 hours). Except for certain preventive services (for which you pay nothing if the doctor or other health care provider accepts assignment), you usually pay 20% of the Medicare-approved amount to both the ambulatory surgical center and the doctor who treats you, and the Part B deductible applies. You pay all of the facility service fees for procedures Medicare doesn't cover in ambulatory surgical centers.

> Get estimated Original Medicare costs of outpatient procedures performed in ambulatory surgical centers by visiting Medicare.gov/procedure-price-lookup.

Behavioral health integration services

If you have a behavioral health condition (like depression, anxiety, or another mental health condition), Medicare may pay for a health care provider's help to manage that condition if your provider offers the Psychiatric Collaborative Care Model. The Psychiatric Collaborative Care Model is a set of integrated behavioral health services that includes care management support if you have a behavioral health condition. This care management support may include:

- Care planning for behavioral health conditions
- Ongoing assessment of your condition
- Medication support
- Counseling
- Other treatment your provider recommends

Your health care provider will ask you to sign an agreement for you to get this set of services on a monthly basis. You pay a monthly fee, and the Part B deductible and coinsurance apply.

Blood

If the provider gets blood from a blood bank at no charge, you won't have to pay for it or replace it. However, you'll pay a copayment for the blood processing and handling services for each unit of blood you get, and the Part B deductible applies. If the provider has to buy blood for you, you must either pay the provider costs for the first 3 units of blood you get in a calendar year, or have the blood donated by you or someone else.

Bone mass measurement (bone density)

This test helps to see if you're at risk for broken bones. It's covered once every 24 months (more often if medically necessary) for people who have certain medical conditions or meet certain criteria. You pay nothing for this test if the doctor or other qualified health care provider accepts assignment.

Breast cancer screening (mammogram)

Medicare covers screening mammograms to check for breast cancer once every 12 months for all women with Medicare who are 40 and older. Medicare covers one baseline mammogram for women between 35–39. You pay nothing for the test if the doctor or other qualified health care provider accepts assignment.

Note: Part B also covers diagnostic mammograms more frequently than once a year when medically necessary. You pay 20% of the Medicare-approved amount for diagnostic mammograms, and the Part B deductible applies.

Cardiac rehabilitation

Medicare covers comprehensive cardiac rehabilitation programs that include exercise, education, and counseling for patients who meet at least one of these conditions:

- A heart attack in the last 12 months
- Coronary artery bypass surgery
- Current stable angina pectoris (chest pain)
- A heart valve repair or replacement
- A coronary angioplasty (a medical procedure used to open a blocked artery) or coronary stenting (a procedure used to keep an artery open)
- A heart or heart-lung transplant
- Stable, chronic heart failure

Medicare also covers intensive cardiac rehabilitation programs that are typically more rigorous or more intense than regular cardiac rehabilitation programs. Services are covered in a doctor's office or hospital outpatient setting. You pay 20% of the Medicare-approved amount if you get the services in a doctor's office. In a hospital outpatient setting, you also pay the hospital a copayment. The Part B deductible applies.

Cardiovascular disease (behavioral therapy)

Medicare will cover one visit per year with a primary care doctor in a primary care setting (like a doctor's office) to help lower your risk for cardiovascular disease. During this visit, the doctor may discuss aspirin use (if appropriate), check your blood pressure, and give you tips to make sure you eat well. You pay nothing if the doctor or other qualified health care provider accepts assignment.

Cardiovascular disease screenings

These screenings include blood tests that help detect conditions that may lead to a heart attack or stroke. Medicare covers these screening tests once every 5 years to test your cholesterol, lipid, lipoprotein, and triglyceride levels. You pay nothing for the tests if the doctor or other qualified health care provider accepts assignment.

Cervical and vaginal cancer screenings

Part B covers Pap tests and pelvic exams to check for cervical and vaginal cancers. As part of the pelvic exam, Medicare also covers a clinical breast exam to check for breast cancer. Medicare covers these screening tests once every 24 months. Medicare covers these screening tests once every 12 months if you're at high risk for cervical or vaginal cancer, or if you're of child-bearing age and had an abnormal Pap test in the past 36 months.

Part B also covers Human Papillomavirus (HPV) tests (when received with a Pap test) once every 5 years if you're 30–65 without HPV symptoms.

You pay nothing for the lab Pap test or for the lab HPV with Pap test if your doctor or other qualified health care provider accepts assignment. You also pay nothing for the Pap test specimen collection and pelvic and breast exams if the doctor or other qualified health care provider accepts assignment.

Chemotherapy

Medicare covers chemotherapy in a doctor's office, freestanding clinic, or hospital outpatient setting for people with cancer. You pay a copayment for chemotherapy in a hospital outpatient setting.

For chemotherapy given in a doctor's office or freestanding clinic, you pay 20% of the Medicare-approved amount, and the Part B deductible applies.

For chemotherapy in a hospital inpatient setting covered under Part A, see Hospital care (inpatient care) on pages 27–28.

Chiropractic services (limited coverage)

Medicare covers manipulation of the spine if medically necessary to correct a subluxation (when one or more of the bones of your spine move out of position) when provided by a chiropractor or other qualified provider. You pay 20% of the Medicare-approved amount, and the Part B deductible applies.

Note: Medicare doesn't cover other services or tests ordered by a chiropractor, including X-rays, massage therapy, and acupuncture. If you think your chiropractor is billing Medicare for chiropractic services that aren't covered, you can report suspected Medicare fraud by calling 1-800-MEDICARE (1-800-633-4227). TTY users can call 1-877-486-2048.

Chronic care management services

If you have 2 or more serious, chronic conditions (like arthritis, asthma, dementia, diabetes, hypertension, heart disease, osteoporosis, and other conditions) that are expected to last at least a year, Medicare may pay for a health care provider's help to manage those conditions. This includes a comprehensive care plan that lists your health problems and goals, other health care providers, medications, community services you have and need, and other information about your health. It also explains the care you need and how your care will be coordinated. Your health care provider will ask you to sign an agreement to provide this service. If you agree, he or she will prepare the care plan, help you with medication management, provide 24/7 access for urgent care needs, give you support when you go from one health care setting to another, review your medicines and how you take them, and help you with other chronic care needs. You pay a monthly fee, and the Part B deductible and coinsurance apply.

Clinical research studies

Clinical research studies test how well different types of medical care work and if they're safe. Medicare covers some costs, like office visits and tests, in qualifying clinical research studies. You may pay 20% of the Medicare-approved amount, and the Part B deductible may apply.

Note: If you're in a Medicare Advantage Plan, some costs may be covered by Original Medicare and some may be covered by your Medicare Advantage Plan.

Colorectal cancer screenings

Medicare covers these screenings to help find precancerous growths or find cancer early, when treatment is most effective. One or more of these tests may be covered:

- **Multi-target stool DNA test**: This lab test is generally covered once every 3 years if you meet all of these conditions:
  - Are between 50–85.
  - Show no signs or symptoms of colorectal disease including, but not limited to, lower gastrointestinal pain, blood in stool, positive guaiac fecal occult blood test or fecal immunochemical test.
  - At average risk for developing colorectal cancer, meaning you:
    - Have no personal history of adenomatous polyps, colorectal cancer, inflammatory bowel disease, including Crohn's Disease and ulcerative colitis.
    - Have no family history of colorectal cancer or adenomatous polyps, familial adenomatous polyposis, or hereditary nonpolyposis colorectal cancer.

You pay nothing for the test if the doctor or other qualified health care provider accepts assignment.

- **Screening fecal occult blood test**: This test is covered once every 12 months if you're 50 or older. You pay nothing for the test if the doctor or other qualified health care provider accepts assignment.
- **Screening flexible sigmoidoscopy**: This test is generally covered once every 48 months if you're 50 or older, or 120 months after a previous screening colonoscopy for those not at high risk. You pay nothing for the test if the doctor or other qualified health care provider accepts assignment.
- **Screening colonoscopy**: This test is generally covered once every 120 months (high risk every 24 months) or 48 months after a previous flexible sigmoidoscopy. There's no minimum age. You pay nothing for the test if the doctor or other qualified health care provider accepts assignment.

  Note: If a polyp or other tissue is found and removed during the colonoscopy, you may have to pay 20% of the Medicare-approved amount for the doctor's services and a copayment in a hospital outpatient setting. The Part B deductible doesn't apply.
- **Screening barium enema**: This test is generally covered once every 48 months if you're 50 or older (high risk every 24 months) when used instead of a sigmoidoscopy or colonoscopy. You pay 20% of the Medicare-approved amount for the doctor services. In a hospital outpatient setting, you also pay the hospital a copayment. The Part B deductible doesn't apply.

Continuous Positive Airway Pressure (CPAP) therapy
Medicare covers a 3-month trial of CPAP therapy if you've been diagnosed with obstructive sleep apnea. Medicare may cover it longer if you meet with your doctor in person, and your doctor documents in your medical record that the CPAP therapy is helping you.

You pay 20% of the Medicare-approved amount for rental of the machine and purchase of related accessories (like masks and tubing), and the Part B deductible applies. Medicare pays the supplier to rent the machine for 13 months if you've been using it without interruption. After you've rented the machine for 13 months, you own it.

Note: If you had a CPAP machine before you got Medicare, Medicare may cover rental or a replacement CPAP machine and/or CPAP accessories if you meet certain requirements.

Defibrillator (implantable automatic)
Medicare covers these devices for some people diagnosed with heart failure. If the surgery takes place in an outpatient setting, you pay 20% of the Medicare-approved amount for the doctor's services. If you get the device as a hospital outpatient, you also pay the hospital a copayment. In most cases, the copayment amount can't be more than the Part A hospital stay deductible. The Part B deductible applies. Part A covers surgeries to implant defibrillators in a hospital inpatient setting. See Hospital care (inpatient care) on pages 27–28.

Depression screening

Medicare covers one depression screening per year. The screening must be done in a primary care setting (like a doctor's office) that can provide follow-up treatment and referrals. You pay nothing for this screening if the doctor or other qualified health care provider accepts assignment.

Diabetes screenings

Medicare covers these screenings if your doctor determines you're at risk for diabetes or diagnosed with prediabetes. You may be eligible for up to 2 diabetes screenings each year. You pay nothing for the test if your doctor or other qualified health care provider accepts assignment.

Medicare Diabetes Prevention Program

Medicare covers a once-per-lifetime health behavior change program to help you prevent type 2 diabetes. The program begins with 16 core sessions offered in a group setting over a 6-month period. In these sessions, you'll get:

- Training to make realistic, lasting behavior changes around diet and exercise
- Tips on how to get more exercise
- Strategies to control your weight
- A coach, specially trained to help keep you motivated
- Support from people with similar goals and challenges

Once you complete the core sessions, you'll get:

- 6 more months of follow-up sessions to help you maintain healthy habits
- An additional 12 months of ongoing maintenance sessions if you meet certain weight loss and attendance goals

To be eligible, you must have:

- Medicare Part B (or a Medicare Advantage Plan)
- A hemoglobin A1c test result between 5.7 and 6.4%, a fasting plasma glucose of 110-125mg/dL, or a 2-hour plasma glucose of 140-199 mg/dL (oral glucose tolerance test) within 12 months prior to attending the first core session
- A body mass index (BMI) of 25 or more (BMI of 23 or more if you're Asian)
- Never been diagnosed with type 1 or type 2 diabetes or End-Stage Renal Disease (ESRD)
- Never participated in the Medicare Diabetes Prevention Program

You pay nothing for these services if you're eligible.

To find a Medicare Diabetes Prevention Program supplier, visit **Medicare.gov/contacts**.

Diabetes self-management training

Medicare covers diabetes outpatient self-management training to teach you to cope with and manage your diabetes. The program may include tips for eating healthy, being active, monitoring blood sugar, taking medication, and reducing risks. You must have diabetes and a written order from your doctor or other qualified health care provider who's treating your diabetes. You pay 20% of the Medicare-approved amount, and the Part B deductible applies.

Diabetes equipment and supplies and therapeutic shoes

Medicare covers blood sugar or glucose testing monitors and infusion pumps, if necessary, to administer insulin and related supplies and accessories for this equipment, including test strips, lancets, glucose sensors, tubing, and insulin. Medicare also covers therapeutic shoes (custom molded or extra depth shoes) and inserts for these shoes. You pay 20% of the Medicare-approved amount, and the Part B deductible applies.

Note: Medicare prescription drug coverage (Part D) may cover insulin, certain medical supplies used to inject insulin (like syringes), disposable pumps, and some oral diabetes drugs. Check with your plan for more information.

Doctor and other health care provider services

Medicare covers medically necessary doctor services (including outpatient services and some doctor services you get when you're a hospital inpatient) and covered preventive services. Medicare also covers services provided by other health care providers, like physician assistants, nurse practitioners, clinical nurse specialists, certified nurse-midwives, clinical social workers, physical therapists, and clinical psychologists. Except for certain preventive services (for which you may pay nothing), you pay 20% of the Medicare-approved amount, and the Part B deductible applies.

Durable medical equipment (DME)

Medicare covers items like oxygen and oxygen equipment, wheelchairs, walkers, and hospital beds ordered by a doctor or other health care provider enrolled in Medicare for use in the home. Some items must be rented. You pay 20% of the Medicare-approved amount, and the Part B deductible applies.

Make sure your doctors and DME suppliers are enrolled in Medicare.
Doctors and suppliers have to meet strict standards to enroll and stay enrolled in Medicare. If your doctors or suppliers aren't enrolled, Medicare won't pay the claims they submit. It's also important to ask your suppliers if they participate in Medicare before you get DME. If suppliers are participating suppliers, they must accept assignment (that is, they're limited to charging you only coinsurance and the Part B deductible for the Medicare-approved amount). If suppliers aren't participating and don't accept assignment, there's no limit on the amount they can charge you. To find suppliers who accept assignment, visit **Medicare.gov/supplierdirectory** or call 1-800-MEDICARE (1-800-633-4227). TTY users can call 1-877-486-2048. You can also call 1-800-MEDICARE if you're having problems with your DME supplier, or you need to file a complaint.

For more information, visit **Medicare.gov/publications** to view the booklet "Medicare Coverage of Durable Medical Equipment and Other Devices."

EKG or ECG (electrocardiogram) screening

Medicare covers a one-time screening EKG/ECG if referred by your doctor or other health care provider as part of your one-time "Welcome to Medicare" preventive visit. See page 48. You pay 20% of the Medicare-approved amount, and the Part B deductible applies. An EKG/ECG is also covered as a diagnostic test. See page 47. If you have the test at a hospital or a hospital-owned clinic, you also pay the hospital a copayment.

Emergency department services

These services are covered when you have an injury, a sudden illness, or an illness that quickly gets much worse. You pay a specified copayment for the hospital emergency department visit, and you pay 20% of the Medicare-approved amount for the doctor's or other health care provider's services. The Part B deductible applies. However, your costs may be different if you're admitted to the hospital as an inpatient.

Eyeglasses (after cataract surgery)

Medicare covers one pair of eyeglasses with standard frames (or one set of contact lenses) after each cataract surgery that implants an intraocular lens. You pay 20% of the Medicare-approved amount, and the Part B deductible applies.

Note: Medicare will only pay for contact lenses or eyeglasses provided by a supplier enrolled in Medicare, no matter who submits the claim (you or your provider).

Federally Qualified Health Center (FQHC) services

FQHCs provide many outpatient primary care and preventive health services. There's no deductible, and generally, you're responsible for paying 20% of the charges. You pay nothing for most preventive services. All FQHCs offer discounts if your income is limited. To find an FQHC near you, visit **findahealthcenter.hrsa.gov**.

 ### Flu shots

Medicare covers one flu shot (or vaccine) per flu season. You pay nothing for the flu shot if the doctor or other qualified health care provider accepts assignment for giving the shot.

Foot exams and treatment

Medicare covers foot exams and treatment if you have diabetes-related nerve damage and/or meet certain conditions. You pay 20% of the Medicare-approved amount, and the Part B deductible applies. In a hospital outpatient setting, you also pay the hospital a copayment.

Glaucoma tests

These tests are covered once every 12 months for people at high risk for the eye disease glaucoma. You're at high risk if you have diabetes, a family history of glaucoma, are African American and 50 or older, or are Hispanic and 65 or older. An eye doctor who's legally allowed by the state must do the tests. You pay 20% of the Medicare-approved amount, and the Part B deductible applies. In a hospital outpatient setting, you also pay the hospital a copayment.

Hearing and balance exams

Medicare covers these exams if your doctor or other health care provider orders them to see if you need medical treatment. You pay 20% of the Medicare-approved amount, and the Part B deductible applies. In a hospital outpatient setting, you also pay the hospital a copayment.

Note: Original Medicare doesn't cover hearing aids or exams for fitting hearing aids.

Hepatitis B shots

Medicare covers these shots (or vaccines) for people at medium or high risk for Hepatitis B. Some risk factors include hemophilia, End-Stage Renal Disease (ESRD), diabetes, if you live with someone who has Hepatitis B, or if you're a health care worker and have frequent contact with blood or body fluids. Check with your doctor to see if you're at medium or high risk for Hepatitis B. You pay nothing for the shot if the doctor or other qualified health care provider accepts assignment.

Hepatitis B Virus (HBV) infection screening

Medicare covers HBV infection screenings if you meet one of these conditions:

- You're at high risk for HBV infection.
- You're pregnant.

Medicare will only cover HBV infection screenings if they're ordered by a primary care provider.

HBV infection screenings are covered:

- Annually only for those with continued high risk who don't get a Hepatitis B vaccination.
- For pregnant women:
  - At the first prenatal visit for each pregnancy.
  - At the time of delivery for those with new or continued risk factors.
  - At the first prenatal visit for future pregnancies, even if you previously got the Hepatitis B shot or had negative HBV screening results.

You pay nothing for the screening test if the doctor or other qualified health care provider accepts assignment.

Hepatitis C screening test
Medicare covers one Hepatitis C screening test if you meet one of these conditions:

- You're at high risk because you have a current or past history of illicit injection drug use.
- You had a blood transfusion before 1992.
- You were born between 1945–1965.

Medicare also covers yearly repeat screenings for certain people at high risk.

Medicare will only cover Hepatitis C screening tests if they're ordered by your health care provider. You pay nothing for the screening test if the doctor or other qualified health care provider accepts assignment.

HIV (Human Immunodeficiency Virus) screening
Medicare covers HIV screenings once every 12 months if you're:

- Between 15–65.
- Younger than 15 and older than 65, and at increased risk.

Medicare also covers this test up to 3 times during a pregnancy.

You pay nothing for the HIV screening if the doctor or other qualified health care provider accepts assignment.

Home health services
Medicare covers home health benefits under Part A and/or Part B. Medicare covers medically necessary part-time or intermittent skilled nursing care, and/or physical therapy, speech-language pathology services, or continued occupational therapy services. A doctor, or certain health care professionals who work with a doctor, must see you face-to-face before a doctor can certify that you need home health services. A doctor must order your care, and a Medicare-certified home health agency must provide it.

Home health services may also include medical social services, part-time or intermittent home health aide services, durable medical equipment, and medical supplies for use at home. You must be "homebound," which means:

- You have trouble leaving your home without help (like using a cane, wheelchair, walker, or crutches; special transportation; or help from another person) because of an illness or injury.
- Leaving your home isn't recommended because of your condition.
- You're normally unable to leave your home because it's a major effort.

You pay nothing for covered home health services. However, for Medicare-covered durable medical equipment, you pay 20% of the Medicare-approved amount, and the Part B deductible applies.

Kidney dialysis services and supplies

Generally, Medicare covers 3 dialysis treatments per week if you have End-Stage Renal Disease (ESRD). This includes most ESRD-related drugs and biological products, and all laboratory tests, home dialysis training, support services, equipment, and supplies. The dialysis facility is responsible for coordinating your dialysis services (at home or in a facility). You pay 20% of the Medicare-approved amount, and the Part B deductible applies.

Kidney disease education services

Medicare covers up to 6 sessions of kidney disease education services if you have Stage IV chronic kidney disease, and your doctor or other health care provider refers you for the service. You pay 20% of the Medicare-approved amount, and the Part B deductible applies.

Laboratory services

Medicare covers laboratory services including certain blood tests, urinalysis, certain tests on tissue specimens, and some screening tests. You generally pay nothing for these services.

Lung cancer screening

Medicare covers a lung cancer screening with Low Dose Computed Tomography (LDCT) once per year if you meet all of these conditions:

- You're 55–77.
- You're asymptomatic (don't have signs or symptoms of lung cancer).
- You're either a current smoker or have quit smoking within the last 15 years.
- You have a tobacco smoking history of at least 30 "pack years" (an average of one pack a day for 30 years).
- You get a written order from a doctor or other qualified health care provider.

You generally pay nothing for this service if the health care provider accepts assignment.

Note: Before your first lung cancer screening, you'll need to schedule an appointment with your doctor to discuss the benefits and risks of lung cancer screening. You and your doctor can decide whether a lung cancer screening is right for you.

Medical nutrition therapy services

Medicare covers medical nutrition therapy (MNT) services if you have diabetes or kidney disease, or you've had a kidney transplant in the last 36 months, and your doctor refers you for services. MNT services are furnished only by Registered Dietitians (RDs) or nutrition professionals who meet certain requirements. You pay nothing for these preventive services because the deductible and coinsurance don't apply.

Mental health care (outpatient)

Medicare covers mental health care services to help with conditions like depression and anxiety. Coverage includes services generally provided in an outpatient setting (like a doctor's or other health care provider's office, or hospital outpatient department), including visits with a psychiatrist or other doctor, clinical psychologist, nurse practitioner, physician assistant, clinical nurse specialist, or clinical social worker. Covered mental health care includes Partial Hospitalization Program (PHP) services, which is intensive outpatient mental health day treatment. PHP services are provided by a hospital to its outpatients or by a community mental health center.

Generally, you pay 20% of the Medicare-approved amount and the Part B deductible applies for mental health care services.

Note: Inpatient mental health care is covered under Part A.

Obesity screening and counseling

If you have a body mass index (BMI) of 30 or more, Medicare covers face-to-face individual behavioral therapy sessions to help you lose weight. This counseling is covered if you get it in a primary care setting (like a doctor's office), where it can be coordinated with your other care and a personalized prevention plan. You pay nothing for this service if the doctor or other qualified health care provider accepts assignment.

Occupational therapy

Medicare covers evaluation and treatment to help you perform activities of daily living (like dressing or bathing) to maintain current capabilities or slow decline when your doctor or other health care provider certifies you need it. You pay 20% of the Medicare-approved amount, and the Part B deductible applies.

Opioid use disorder treatment services

Starting January 1, 2020, Medicare will cover opioid use disorder treatment services provided by opioid treatment programs. The services will include medication, counseling, drug testing, and individual and group therapy. Counseling and therapy services will be covered in person and by virtual delivery (using 2-way audio/video communication technology). Under Original Medicare, you will pay nothing for these services if you get them from an opioid treatment provider who's enrolled in Medicare. Talk to your doctor or other health care provider to find out where you can go for these services.

Outpatient hospital services

Medicare covers many diagnostic and treatment services in hospital outpatient departments. Generally, you pay 20% of the Medicare-approved amount for the doctor's or other health care provider's services. You may pay more for services you get in a hospital outpatient setting than you'll pay for the same care in a doctor's office. In addition to the amount you pay the doctor, you'll also usually pay the hospital a copayment for each service you get in a hospital outpatient setting, except for certain preventive services that don't have a copayment. In most cases, the copayment can't be more than the Part A hospital stay deductible for each service. The Part B deductible applies, except for certain preventive services. If you get hospital outpatient services in a critical access hospital, your copayment may be higher and may exceed the Part A hospital stay deductible.

> Get estimated costs of outpatient procedures performed in hospital outpatient departments by visiting **Medicare.gov/procedure-price-lookup**.

Outpatient medical and surgical services and supplies

Medicare covers approved procedures like X-rays, casts, stitches, or outpatient surgeries. You pay 20% of the Medicare-approved amount for the doctor's or other health care provider's services. You generally pay the hospital a copayment for each service you get in a hospital outpatient setting. In most cases, for each service provided, the copayment can't be more than the Part A hospital stay deductible. The Part B deductible applies, and you pay all costs for items or services that Medicare doesn't cover.

Physical therapy

Medicare covers evaluation and treatment for injuries and diseases that change your ability to function, or to maintain current function or slow decline, when your doctor or other health care provider certifies your need for it. You pay 20% of the Medicare-approved amount, and the Part B deductible applies.

Pneumococcal shots

Medicare covers pneumococcal shots (or vaccines) to help prevent pneumococcal infections (like certain types of pneumonia). The two shots are the 23-valent pneumococcal polysaccharide vaccine (PPSV23) and 13-valent pneumococcal conjugate vaccine (PCV13). The two shots protect against different strains of the bacteria. Medicare covers the first shot at any time, and also covers a different second shot if it's given one year (or later) after the first shot. Talk with your doctor or other health care provider to see if you need one or both of the pneumococcal shots. You pay nothing for these shots if the doctor or other qualified health care provider accepts assignment for giving the shots.

Prescription drugs (limited)

Medicare covers a limited number of drugs like injections you get in a doctor's office, certain oral anti-cancer drugs, drugs used with some types of durable medical equipment (like a nebulizer or external infusion pump), immunosuppressant drugs (see page 47), and, under very limited circumstances, certain drugs you get in a hospital outpatient setting. You pay 20% of the Medicare-approved amount for these covered drugs, and the Part B deductible applies.

If the covered drugs you get in a hospital outpatient setting are part of your outpatient services, you pay a copayment for the services. However, other types of drugs in a hospital outpatient setting (sometimes called "self-administered drugs" or drugs you'd normally take on your own) aren't covered by Part B. What you pay depends on whether you have Part D or other prescription drug coverage, whether your drug plan covers the drug, and whether the hospital's pharmacy is in your drug plan's network. Contact your prescription drug plan to find out what you pay for drugs you get in a hospital outpatient setting that aren't covered under Part B.

Other than the examples above, you pay 100% for most prescription drugs, unless you have Part D or other drug coverage. See pages 73–82 for more information about Part D.

Prostate cancer screenings

Medicare covers a Prostate Specific Antigen (PSA) test and a digital rectal exam once every 12 months for men over 50 (beginning the day after your 50th birthday). You pay nothing for the PSA test. For the digital rectal exam, you pay 20% of the Medicare-approved amount, and the Part B deductible applies. In a hospital outpatient setting, you also pay the hospital a copayment.

Prosthetic/orthotic items

Medicare covers arm, leg, back, and neck braces; artificial eyes; artificial limbs (and their replacement parts); and prosthetic devices needed to replace an internal body organ or function of the organ (including ostomy supplies, parenteral and enteral nutrition therapy, and some types of breast prostheses after a mastectomy) when ordered by a doctor or other health care provider enrolled in Medicare.

For Medicare to cover your prosthetic or orthotic, you must go to a supplier that's enrolled in Medicare. You pay 20% of the Medicare-approved amount, and the Part B deductible applies.

Pulmonary rehabilitation

Medicare covers a comprehensive pulmonary rehabilitation program if you have moderate to very severe chronic obstructive pulmonary disease (COPD) and have a referral from the doctor treating this chronic respiratory disease. You pay 20% of the Medicare-approved amount if you get the service in a doctor's office. You also pay the hospital a copayment per session if you get the service in a hospital outpatient setting. The Part B deductible applies.

Rural Health Clinic (RHC) services

RHCs furnish many outpatient primary care and preventive health services. RHCs are located in rural and underserved areas. Generally, you're responsible for paying 20% of the charges, and the Part B deductible applies. You pay nothing for most preventive services.

Second surgical opinions

Medicare covers second surgical opinions for surgery that isn't an emergency. In some cases, Medicare covers third surgical opinions. You pay 20% of the Medicare-approved amount, and the Part B deductible applies.

Sexually transmitted infection (STI) screening and counseling

Medicare covers STI screenings for chlamydia, gonorrhea, syphilis, and Hepatitis B. These screenings are covered if you're pregnant or at increased risk for an STI when the tests are ordered by a primary care provider. Medicare covers these tests once every 12 months or at certain times during pregnancy.

Medicare also covers up to 2 individual, 20–30 minute, face-to-face, high-intensity behavioral counseling sessions each year for sexually active adults at increased risk for STIs. Medicare will only cover these counseling sessions if they're provided by a primary care doctor or other primary care provider and take place in a primary care setting (like a doctor's office). Counseling conducted in an inpatient setting, like a skilled nursing facility, won't be covered as a preventive service.

You pay nothing for these services if the primary care doctor or other qualified health care provider accepts assignment.

Shots (or vaccines)

Part B covers:

- Yearly flu shots. See page 38.
- Hepatitis B shots. See page 39.
- Pneumococcal shots. See page 43.

Note about Part D coverage: Part D covers all other recommended adult immunizations (for example the shingles and TDAP (Tetanus, diphtheria, and pertussis) vaccines) to prevent illness. Talk to your provider about which ones are right for you.

Smoking and tobacco-use cessation (counseling to prevent tobacco use & tobacco-caused disease)

Medicare covers up to 8 face-to-face visits in a 12-month period. All people with Medicare who use tobacco are covered. You pay nothing for the counseling sessions if the doctor or other qualified health care provider accepts assignment.

Speech-language pathology services

Medicare covers evaluation and treatment to regain and strengthen speech and language skills, including cognitive and swallowing skills, or to maintain current function or slow decline, when your doctor or other health care provider certifies you need it. You pay 20% of the Medicare-approved amount, and the Part B deductible applies.

Surgical dressing services

Medicare covers medically necessary treatment of a surgical or surgically treated wound. You pay 20% of the Medicare-approved amount for the doctor's or other health care provider's services. You pay a fixed copayment for these services when you get them in a hospital outpatient setting. The Part B deductible applies. You pay nothing for the supplies.

Telehealth

Medicare covers services like office visits, psychotherapy, consultations, and certain other medical or health services provided by an eligible provider who isn't at your location using an interactive, two-way telecommunications system (like real-time audio and video). These services are available in rural areas, under certain conditions, but only if you're located at: a doctor's office, hospital, critical access hospital, Rural Health Clinic, Federally Qualified Health Center, hospital-based dialysis facility, skilled nursing facility, or community mental health center.

Medicare has made these changes to telehealth in 2019:

- You can get certain telehealth services at renal dialysis facilities and at home.
- You can get telehealth services for faster diagnosis, evaluation, or treatment of symptoms of an acute stroke no matter where you're located.
- If you have a substance use disorder or a co-occurring mental health disorder, you can get telehealth services from home.

For most of these services, you'll pay the same amount that you would if you got the services in person.

Starting in 2020, Medicare Advantage Plans may offer more telehealth benefits than Original Medicare. These benefits will be available no matter where you're located, and you can use them at home instead of going to a health care facility. Check with your plan to see what additional telehealth benefits are offered.

Tests (other than lab tests)

Medicare covers X-rays, MRIs, CT scans, EKG/ECGs, and some other diagnostic tests. You pay 20% of the Medicare-approved amount, and the Part B deductible applies. If you get the test at a hospital as an outpatient, you also pay the hospital a copayment that may be more than 20% of the Medicare-approved amount, but, in most cases, this amount can't be more than the Part A hospital stay deductible. See Laboratory services on page 40 for other Part B-covered tests.

Transitional care management services

Medicare may cover this service if you're returning to your community after a stay at certain facilities, like a hospital or skilled nursing facility. The health care provider who's managing your transition back into the community will work to coordinate and manage your care for the first 30 days after you return home. He or she will work with you, your family, and caregiver(s), as appropriate, and other health care providers. You'll also be able to get an in-person office visit within 2 weeks of your return home. The health care provider may also review information on the care you received in the facility, provide information to help you transition back to living at home, work with other care providers, help you with referrals or arrangements for follow-up care or community resources, assist you with scheduling, and help you manage your medications. The Part B deductible and coinsurance apply.

Transplants and immunosuppressive drugs

Medicare covers doctor services for heart, lung, kidney, pancreas, intestine, and liver transplants under certain conditions but only in Medicare-certified facilities. Medicare also covers bone marrow and cornea transplants under certain conditions.

Note: The transplant surgery may be covered as a hospital inpatient service under Part A. See pages 27–28 for more information.

Medicare covers immunosuppressive drugs if the transplant was covered by Medicare or an employer or union group health plan was required to pay before Medicare paid for the transplant. You must have Part A at the time of the covered transplant, and you must have Part B at the time you get immunosuppressive drugs. You pay 20% of the Medicare-approved amount for the drugs, and the Part B deductible applies.

If you're thinking about joining a Medicare Advantage Plan and are on a transplant waiting list or believe you need a transplant, check with the plan before you join to make sure your doctors, other health care providers, and hospitals are in the plan's network. Also, check the plan's coverage rules for prior authorization.

Note: Medicare drug plans (Part D) may cover immunosuppressive drugs if they aren't covered by Original Medicare.

Medicare pays the full cost of care for your kidney donor. You and your donor won't have to pay a deductible, coinsurance, or any other costs for their hospital stay.

Travel (health care needed when traveling outside the U.S.)

Medicare generally doesn't cover health care while you're traveling outside the U.S. (The "U.S." includes the 50 states, the District of Columbia, Puerto Rico, the U.S. Virgin Islands, Guam, the Northern Mariana Islands, and American Samoa.) There are some exceptions, including cases where Medicare may pay for services you get while on board a ship within the territorial waters adjoining the land areas of the U.S. Medicare may pay for inpatient hospital, doctor, or ambulance services you get in a foreign country in these rare cases:

- You're in the U.S. when an emergency occurs, and the foreign hospital is closer than the nearest U.S. hospital that can treat your medical condition.
- You're traveling through Canada without unreasonable delay by the most direct route between Alaska and another U.S. state when a medical emergency occurs, and the Canadian hospital is closer than the nearest U.S. hospital that can treat the emergency.
- You live in the U.S. and the foreign hospital is closer to your home than the nearest U.S. hospital that can treat your medical condition, regardless of whether an emergency exists.

Medicare may cover medically necessary ambulance transportation to a foreign hospital only with admission for medically necessary covered inpatient hospital services. You pay 20% of the Medicare-approved amount, and the Part B deductible applies.

Urgently needed care

Medicare covers urgently needed care to treat a sudden illness or injury that isn't a medical emergency. You pay 20% of the Medicare-approved amount for the doctor's or other health care provider's services, and the Part B deductible applies. In a hospital outpatient setting, you also pay the hospital a copayment.

"Welcome to Medicare" preventive visit

During the first 12 months that you have Part B, you can get a "Welcome to Medicare" preventive visit. The visit includes a review of your medical and social history related to your health. It also includes education and counseling about preventive services, including certain screenings, shots or vaccines (like flu, pneumococcal, and other recommended shots or vaccines), and referrals for other care, if needed. When you make your appointment, let your doctor's office know that you'd like to schedule your "Welcome to Medicare" preventive visit. You pay nothing for the "Welcome to Medicare" preventive visit if the doctor or other qualified health care provider accepts assignment.

Important! If your doctor or other health care provider performs additional tests or services during the same visit that aren't covered under this preventive benefit, you may have to pay coinsurance, and the Part B deductible may apply. If the additional tests or services aren't covered by Medicare (for example a routine physical exam), you may have to pay the full amount.

Yearly "Wellness" visit

If you've had Part B for longer than 12 months, you can get a yearly "Wellness" visit to develop or update a personalized plan to prevent disease or disability based on your current health and risk factors. Your provider may also perform a cognitive impairment assessment to look for signs of Alzheimer's disease or dementia. **The yearly "Wellness" visit isn't a physical exam.** This visit is covered once every 12 months.

Your provider will ask you to fill out a questionnaire, called a "Health Risk Assessment," as part of this visit. Answering these questions can help you and your provider develop a personalized prevention plan to help you stay healthy and get the most out of your visit. Your visit should also include a review of preventive services including education and counseling on screenings and recommended shots or vaccines as well as referrals for other care, if needed. When you make your appointment, let your doctor's office know that you'd like to schedule your yearly "Wellness" visit.

Note: Your first yearly "Wellness" visit can't take place within 12 months of your enrollment in Part B or your "Welcome to Medicare" preventive visit. However, you don't need to have had a "Welcome to Medicare" preventive visit to qualify for a yearly "Wellness" visit.

You pay nothing for the yearly "Wellness" visit if the doctor or other qualified health care provider accepts assignment.

Important! If your doctor or other health care provider performs additional tests or services during the same visit that aren't covered under this preventive benefit, you may have to pay coinsurance, and the Part B deductible may apply. If the additional tests or services aren't covered by Medicare (for example a routine physical exam), you may have to pay the full amount.

What's NOT covered by Part A and Part B?

Medicare doesn't cover everything. If you need certain services that aren't covered under Medicare Part A or Part B, you'll have to pay for them yourself unless:

- You have other coverage (including Medicaid) to cover the costs.
- You're in a Medicare Advantage Plan that covers these services.

Some of the items and services that Original Medicare doesn't cover include:
- ✖ Most dental care.
- ✖ Eye exams related to prescribing glasses.
- ✖ Dentures.
- ✖ Cosmetic surgery.
- ✖ Massage therapy.
- ✖ Routine physical exams.
- ✖ Acupuncture.
- ✖ Hearing aids and exams for fitting them.
- ✖ Long-term care. See the next page for more information.
- ✖ Concierge care (also called concierge medicine, retainer-based medicine, boutique medicine, platinum practice, or direct care).

Paying for long-term care

Long-term care (sometimes called "long-term services and supports") includes non-medical care for people who have a chronic illness or disability. This includes non-skilled personal care assistance, like help with everyday activities, including dressing, bathing, using the bathroom, home-delivered meals, adult day health care, and other services. **Medicare and most health insurance plans, including Medicare Supplement Insurance (Medigap) policies, don't pay for this type of care, sometimes called "custodial care."** You may be eligible for this type of care through Medicaid, or you can choose to buy private long-term care insurance.

Long-term care can be provided at home, in the community, in an assisted living facility, or in a nursing home. It's important to start planning for long-term care now to maintain your independence and to make sure you get the care you may need, in the setting you want, now and in the future.

Long-term care resources

Use these resources to get more information about long-term care:

- Visit longtermcare.gov to learn more about planning for long-term care.
- Call your State Insurance Department to get information about long-term care insurance. Visit Medicare.gov/contacts, or call 1-800-MEDICARE (1-800-633-4227) to get the phone number. TTY users can call 1-877-486-2048.
- Call your Medicaid office (State Medical Assistance Office), and ask for information about long-term care coverage. To get the phone number for your state, visit Medicare.gov/contacts. You can also call 1-800-MEDICARE.
- Get a copy of "A Shopper's Guide to Long-Term Care Insurance" from the National Association of Insurance Commissioners at naic.org/documents/prod_serv_consumer_ltc_lp.pdf.
- Call your State Health Insurance Assistance Program (SHIP). See pages 109–112 for the phone number.
- Visit the Eldercare Locator, a public service of the U.S. Administration on Aging, at eldercare.acl.gov to find help in your community.

Special Needs Plans (SNPs) are a type of Medicare Advantage Plan that may be able to cover long-term care if you have Medicare and Medicaid. See page 64 to learn more about SNPs. Also, some Medicare Advantage Plans may cover certain extra benefits, like adult day-care services. See page 56.

SECTION 3

Original Medicare

How does Original Medicare work?

Original Medicare is one of your health coverage choices as part of Medicare. You'll have Original Medicare unless you choose a Medicare Advantage Plan or other type of Medicare health plan.

You generally have to pay a portion of the cost for each service covered by Original Medicare. See the next page for the general rules about how it works.

Original Medicare

Can I get my health care from any doctor, other health care provider, or hospital?	In most cases, yes. You can go to any doctor, other health care provider, hospital, or other facility that's enrolled in Medicare and accepting Medicare patients. Visit Medicare.gov to search for and compare health care providers, hospitals, and facilities in your area.
Are prescription drugs covered?	No, with a few exceptions (see pages 26–27, 41, and 43), most prescriptions aren't covered. You can add drug coverage by joining a Medicare Prescription Drug Plan (Part D). See pages 73–82.
Do I need to choose a primary care doctor?	No.
Do I have to get a referral to see a specialist?	In most cases, no, but the specialist must be enrolled in Medicare.
Should I get a supplemental policy?	You may already have employer or union coverage that may pay costs that Original Medicare doesn't. If not, you may want to buy a Medicare Supplement Insurance (Medigap) policy if you're eligible. See pages 69–72.

★ **Note:** Definitions of blue words are on pages 113–116.

What else do I need to know about Original Medicare?	• You generally pay a set amount for your health care (deductible) before Medicare pays its share. Once Medicare pays its share, you pay a coinsurance or copayment for covered services and supplies. **There's no yearly limit for what you pay out-of-pocket.**
	• You usually pay a monthly premium for Part B.
	• You generally don't need to file Medicare claims. Providers and suppliers must file your claims for the covered services and supplies you get.

What do I pay?

Your out-of-pocket costs in Original Medicare depend on:

• Whether you have Part A and/or Part B. Most people have both.
• Whether your doctor, other health care provider, or supplier accepts "assignment." See the next page for more information.
• The type of health care you need and how often you need it.
• If you choose to get services or supplies Medicare doesn't cover, you pay all costs unless you have other insurance that covers them.
• Whether you have other health insurance that works with Medicare.
• Whether you have Medicaid or get help from your state paying your Medicare costs.
• Whether you have a Medicare Supplement Insurance (Medigap) policy.
• Whether you and your doctor or other health care provider sign a private contract. See page 54.

How do I know what Medicare paid?

If you have Original Medicare, you'll get a "Medicare Summary Notice" (MSN) in the mail every 3 months that lists all the services billed to Medicare. The MSN shows what Medicare paid and what you may owe the provider. The MSN isn't a bill. Review your MSNs to be sure you got all the services, supplies, or equipment listed. If you disagree with a decision by Medicare not to pay for (cover) a service, the MSN will tell you how to appeal. See page 91 for information on how to file an appeal.

If you need to change your address on your MSN, call Social Security at 1-800-772-1213. TTY users can call 1-800-325-0778. If you get Railroad Retirement Board (RRB) benefits, call the RRB at 1-877-772-5772. TTY users can call 1-312-751-4701.

Your MSN will tell you if you're enrolled in the Qualified Medicare Beneficiary Program (QMB). If you're in the QMB Program, Medicare providers aren't allowed to bill you for Medicare Part A and/or Part B deductibles, coinsurance, or copayments. For more information about QMB and steps to take if you get billed for these costs, see page 86.

Important! ▶ **Get your Medicare Summary Notices electronically**
Go paperless and get your "Medicare Summary Notices" electronically (also called "eMSNs"). You can sign up by visiting MyMedicare.gov. If you sign up for eMSNs, we'll send you an email each month when they're available in your MyMedicare.gov account. The eMSNs contain the same information as paper MSNs. You won't get printed copies of your MSNs in the mail if you choose eMSNs.

> A growing number of computer and mobile applications are connected to Medicare through Blue Button 2.0. If you agree to share your information with one of these applications, it can show you the details of the claims that Medicare has paid on your behalf. See page 103 for more information.

What's assignment?

Assignment means that your doctor, provider, or supplier agrees (or is required by law) to accept the Medicare-approved amount as full payment for covered services.

If your doctor, provider, or supplier accepts assignment:

- Your out-of-pocket costs may be less.
- They agree to charge you only the Medicare deductible and coinsurance amount and usually wait for Medicare to pay its share before asking you to pay your share.
- They have to submit your claim directly to Medicare and can't charge you for submitting the claim.

Non-participating providers haven't signed an agreement to accept assignment for all Medicare-covered services, but they can still choose to accept assignment for individual services. These providers are called "non-participating." Here's what happens if your doctor, provider, or supplier doesn't accept assignment:

- **You might have to pay the entire charge at the time of service.** Your doctor, provider, or supplier is supposed to submit a claim to Medicare for any Medicare-covered services they provide to you. If they don't submit the Medicare claim once you ask them to, call 1-800-MEDICARE (1-800-633-4227). TTY users can call 1-877-486-2048.
- **They can charge you more than the Medicare-approved amount, but there's a limit called "the limiting charge."**

> If you have Original Medicare, you can see any provider you want that takes Medicare, anywhere in the U.S.

What are private contracts?

Certain doctors and other health care providers who don't want to engage with the Medicare program may "opt out" of Medicare. You can still see these providers, but they must enter into a private contract with you (unless you're in need of emergency or urgently needed care). **Medicare won't pay for any services you get under a private contract, so you'll pay the provider's entire charge out of your own pocket.** You and your provider will set up your own payment terms through the private contract. Visit data.cms.gov/opt-out-affidavits to find an "opt out" provider. You can look up a provider by their National Provider Identifier (NPI), or by first and last name.

> To find out if someone accepts assignment or participates in Medicare, visit Medicare.gov/physician or Medicare.gov/supplier. Or, you can call 1-800-MEDICARE. Contact your State Health Insurance Assistance Program (SHIP) to get free help with these topics. See pages 109–112 for the phone number.

SECTION 4

Medicare Advantage Plans & other options

What are Medicare Advantage Plans?

A Medicare Advantage Plan is another way to get your Medicare coverage. Medicare Advantage Plans, sometimes called "Part C" or "MA Plans," are offered by Medicare-approved private companies that must follow rules set by Medicare. If you join a Medicare Advantage Plan, you'll still have Medicare but you'll get most of your Medicare Part A (Hospital Insurance) and Medicare Part B (Medical Insurance) coverage from the Medicare Advantage Plan, not Original Medicare. Most plans include Medicare prescription drug coverage (Part D). In most cases, you'll need to use health care providers who participate in the plan's network. However, many plans offer out-of-network coverage, but sometimes at a higher cost. Remember, you must use the card from your Medicare Advantage Plan to get your Medicare-covered services. Keep your red, white, and blue Medicare card in a safe place because you'll need it if you ever switch back to Original Medicare.

What are the different types of Medicare Advantage Plans?

- **Health Maintenance Organization (HMO) plans**: See page 61.
- **Preferred Provider Organization (PPO) plans**: See page 62.
- **Private Fee-for-Service (PFFS) plans**: See page 63.
- **Special Needs Plans (SNPs)**: See page 64.
- **HMO Point-of-Service (HMOPOS) plans**: These are HMO plans that may allow you to get some services out-of-network for a higher copayment or coinsurance.
- **Medical Savings Account (MSA) Plans**: These plans combine a high-deductible health plan with a bank account that the plan selects. The plan deposits money into the account (usually less than the deductible). You can use the money to pay for your health care services during the year. MSA Plans don't offer Medicare drug coverage. If you want drug coverage, you have to join a Medicare Prescription Drug Plan. For more information on MSA Plans, visit Medicare.gov. To find out if an MSA Plan is available in your area, visit Medicare.gov/plan-compare.

⭐ **Note:** Definitions of blue words are on pages 113–116.

Medicare Advantage Plans cover almost all Medicare Part A and Part B benefits

In all types of Medicare Advantage Plans, you're always covered for emergency and urgent care. Medicare Advantage Plans must cover almost all of the medically necessary services that Original Medicare covers. However, if you're in a Medicare Advantage Plan, Original Medicare will still cover the cost for hospice care, some new Medicare benefits, and some costs for clinical research studies.

Important! ▶ ## Plans can offer extra benefits

Most Medicare Advantage Plans offer coverage for things that aren't covered by Original Medicare, like vision, hearing, dental, and wellness programs (like gym memberships). Plans can also cover more extra benefits than they have in the past, including services like transportation to doctor visits, over-the-counter drugs, adult day-care services, and other health-related services that promote your health and wellness. Plans can also tailor their benefit packages to offer these new benefits to certain chronically ill enrollees. These packages will provide benefits customized to treat those conditions. Check with the plan to see what benefits are offered and if you qualify.

Medicare Advantage Plans must follow Medicare's rules

Medicare pays a fixed amount for your coverage each month to the companies offering Medicare Advantage Plans. These companies must follow rules set by Medicare. However, each Medicare Advantage Plan can charge different out-of-pocket costs and have different rules for how you get services (like whether you need a referral to see a specialist or if you have to go to doctors, facilities, or suppliers that belong to the plan's network for non-emergency or non-urgent care). These rules can change each year. The plan must notify you about any changes before the start of the next enrollment year. **Remember, you have the option each year to keep your current plan, choose a different plan, or switch to Original Medicare.** See page 65. Providers can join or leave a plan's provider network anytime during the year. Your plan can also change the providers in the network anytime during the year. If this happens, you may need to choose a new provider. You generally can't change plans during the year if this happens.

Even though the network of providers may change during the year, the plan must still provide access to qualified doctors and specialists. Your plan will make a good faith effort to provide you with at least 30 days' notice that your provider is leaving your plan so you have time to choose a new provider. Your plan will also help you choose a new provider to continue managing your health care needs.

In most cases, you don't need a referral to see a specialist if you have Original Medicare. See page 51.

Important!

Read the information you get from your plan
If you're in a Medicare Advantage Plan, review the "Annual Notice of Change" (ANOC) and "Evidence of Coverage" (EOC) from your plan each year:

- **The ANOC:** Includes any changes in coverage, costs, service area, and more that will be effective starting in January. Your plan will send you a printed copy by September 30.
- **The EOC:** Gives you details about what the plan covers, how much you pay, and more. Your plan will send you a notice (or printed copy) by October 15, which will include information on how to access the EOC electronically or request a printed copy.

If you don't get these important documents, contact your plan.

What should I know about Medicare Advantage Plans?
Who can join?
You must meet these conditions to join a Medicare Advantage Plan:

- You have Part A and Part B.
- You live in the plan's service area.
- You don't have End-Stage Renal Disease (ESRD), except as explained on page 58.

Joining and leaving
- You can join a Medicare Advantage Plan even if you have a pre-existing condition, except for End-Stage Renal Disease (ESRD), for which there are special rules. See page 58.
- **You can only join or leave a Medicare Advantage Plan at certain times during the year.** See pages 65–66.
- Each year, Medicare Advantage Plans can choose to leave Medicare or make changes to the services they cover and what you pay. If the plan decides to stop participating in Medicare, you'll have to join another Medicare Advantage Plan or return to Original Medicare. See page 90.
- Medicare Advantage Plans must follow certain rules when giving you information about how to join their plan. See page 98 for more information about these rules and how to protect your personal information.

Prescription drug coverage
You usually get prescription drug coverage (Part D) through the Medicare Advantage Plan. In certain types of plans that can't offer drug coverage (MSA plans) or choose not to offer drug coverage (certain PFFS plans), you can join a separate Medicare Prescription Drug Plan. **If you're in a Medicare Advantage HMO, HMOPOS, or PPO, and you join a stand-alone Medicare Prescription Drug Plan, you'll be disenrolled from your Medicare Advantage Plan and returned to Original Medicare.**

What if I have other coverage?

Talk to your employer, union, or other benefits administrator about their rules before you join a Medicare Advantage Plan. In some cases, joining a Medicare Advantage Plan might cause you to lose your employer or union coverage for yourself, your spouse, and dependents and you may not be able to get it back. In other cases, if you join a Medicare Advantage Plan, you may still be able to use your employer or union coverage along with the Medicare Advantage Plan you join. Your employer or union may also offer a Medicare Advantage retiree health plan that they sponsor.

What if I have a Medicare Supplement Insurance (Medigap) policy?

You can't enroll in (and don't need) a Medicare Supplement Insurance (Medigap) policy while you're in a Medicare Advantage Plan. You can't use it to pay for any expenses (copayments, deductibles, and premiums) you have under a Medicare Advantage Plan.

> If you already have a Medigap policy and join a Medicare Advantage Plan, you can drop your Medigap policy. **Keep in mind that if you drop your Medigap policy to join a Medicare Advantage Plan, you may not be able to get it back. See page 72.**

What if I have End-Stage Renal Disease (ESRD)?

If you have End-Stage Renal Disease (ESRD), you can only join a Medicare Advantage Plan in certain situations:

- If you're already in a Medicare Advantage Plan when you develop ESRD, you can stay in your plan or you may be able to join another Medicare Advantage Plan offered by the same company.
- If you're in a Medicare Advantage Plan, and the plan leaves Medicare or no longer provides coverage in your area, you have a one-time right to join another Medicare Advantage Plan.
- If you have an employer or union health plan or other health coverage through a company that offers one or more Medicare Advantage Plan(s), you may be able to join one of that company's Medicare Advantage Plans.
- If you're medically determined to no longer have ESRD (for example you've had a successful kidney transplant), you may be able to join a Medicare Advantage Plan.
- You may be able to join a Medicare Special Needs Plan (SNP) that covers people with ESRD if one is available in your area.

Starting in 2021, people with ESRD will be able to join Medicare Advantage Plans without these restrictions.

Note: If you have ESRD and Original Medicare, you may join a Medicare Prescription Drug Plan.

What do I pay?

Your out-of-pocket costs in a Medicare Advantage Plan depend on:

- Whether the plan charges a monthly premium. You pay this in addition to the Part B premium.
- Whether the plan pays any of your monthly Medicare premiums. Some Medicare Advantage Plans will help pay all or part of your Part B premium. This benefit is sometimes called a "Medicare Part B premium reduction."
- Whether the plan has a yearly deductible or any additional deductibles for certain services.
- How much you pay for each visit or service (copayments or coinsurance). Medicare Advantage Plans can't charge more than Original Medicare for certain services, like chemotherapy, dialysis, and skilled nursing facility care.
- The type of health care services you need and how often you get them.
- Whether you get services from a network provider or a provider that doesn't contract with the plan. If you go to a doctor, other health care provider, facility, or supplier that doesn't belong to the plan's network for non-emergency or non-urgent care services, your services may not be covered, or your costs could be higher. In most cases, this applies to Medicare Advantage HMOs and PPOs.
- Whether you go to a doctor or supplier who accepts assignment (if you're in a Preferred Provider Organization, Private Fee-for-Service Plan, or Medical Savings Account Plan and you go out-of-network). See page 53 for more information about assignment.
- Whether the plan offers extra benefits (in addition to Original Medicare benefits) and if you need to pay extra to get them.
- The plan's yearly limit on your out-of-pocket costs for all Part A and Part B medical services. Once you reach this limit, you'll pay nothing for Part A- and Part B-covered services.
- Whether you have Medicaid or get help from your state.

To learn more about your costs in specific Medicare Advantage Plans, visit **Medicare.gov/plan-compare**.

How do I know what's covered?
You can get a decision from your plan in advance to see if a service, drug, or supply is covered. You can also find out how much you'll have to pay. **This is called an "organization determination."** Sometimes you have to do this as prior authorization for the service, drug, or supply to be covered.

You, your representative, or your doctor can request an organization determination. You also have the option to ask for a fast decision, based on your health needs. If your plan denies coverage, the plan must tell you in writing, and you have the right to an appeal. See pages 89–92.

If a plan provider refers you for a service or to a provider outside the network, but doesn't get an organization determination in advance, **this is called "plan directed care."** In most cases you won't have to pay more than the plan's usual cost sharing. Check with your plan for more information about this protection.

Types of Medicare Advantage Plans

 ### Health Maintenance Organization (HMO) plan

Can I get my health care from any doctor, other health care provider, or hospital?
No. You generally must get your care and services from doctors, other health care providers, or hospitals in the plan's network (except emergency care, out-of-area urgent care, or out-of-area dialysis). In some HMO plans, you may be able to go out-of-network for certain services, usually for a higher cost. This is called an HMO with a point-of-service (POS) option.

Are prescription drugs covered?
In most cases, yes. If you want Medicare drug coverage, you must join an HMO plan that offers prescription drug coverage.

Do I need to choose a primary care doctor?
In most cases, yes.

Do I have to get a referral to see a specialist?
In most cases, yes. Certain services, like yearly screening mammograms, don't require a referral.

What else do I need to know about this type of plan?
- If your doctor or other health care provider leaves the plan's network, your plan will notify you. You may choose another doctor in the plan's network.
- If you get health care outside the plan's network, you may have to pay the full cost.
- It's important that you follow the plan's rules, like getting prior approval for a certain service when needed.
- If you need more information than what's listed on this page, check with the plan.

PPO

Preferred Provider Organization (PPO) plan

Can I get my health care from any doctor, other health care provider, or hospital?
Yes. PPO plans have network doctors, other health care providers, and hospitals, but you can also use out-of-network providers for covered services, usually for a higher cost. You're always covered for emergency and urgent care.

Are prescription drugs covered?
In most cases, yes. If you want Medicare drug coverage, you must join a PPO plan that offers prescription drug coverage.

Do I need to choose a primary care doctor?
No.

Do I have to get a referral to see a specialist?
In most cases, no.

What else do I need to know about this type of plan?
- Because certain providers are "preferred" (as the name suggests), you can save money by using them.
- If you need more information than what's listed on this page, check with the plan.

Private Fee-for-Service (PFFS) plan

Can I get my health care from any doctor, other health care provider, or hospital?

You can go to any Medicare-approved doctor, other health care provider, or hospital that accepts the plan's payment terms and agrees to treat you. If you join a PFFS plan that has a network, you can also see any of the network providers who have agreed to always treat plan members. You can also choose an out-of-network doctor, hospital, or other provider who accepts the plan's terms, but you may pay more.

Are prescription drugs covered?

Sometimes. If your PFFS plan doesn't offer drug coverage, you can join a Medicare Prescription Drug Plan to get coverage.

Do I need to choose a primary care doctor?

No.

Do I have to get a referral to see a specialist?

No.

What else do I need to know about this type of plan?

- The plan decides how much you pay for services. The plan will tell you about your cost sharing in the "Annual Notice of Change" (ANOC) and "Evidence of Coverage" (EOC) documents that it sends each year.
- Some PFFS plans contract with a network of providers who agree to always treat you, even if you've never seen them before.
- Out-of-network doctors, hospitals, and other providers may decide not to treat you, even if you've seen them before.
- For each service you get, make sure to show your plan member card before you get treated.
- In a medical emergency, doctors, hospitals, and other providers must treat you.
- If you need more information than what's listed on this page, check with the plan.

Special Needs Plan (SNP)

> A Special Needs Plan (SNP) provides benefits and services to people with specific diseases, certain health care needs, or limited incomes. SNPs tailor their benefits, provider choices, and drug formularies to best meet the specific needs of the groups they serve.

Can I get my health care from any doctor, other health care provider, or hospital?

Some SNPs cover services out-of-network and some don't. Check with the plan to see if they cover services out-of-network, and if so, how it affects your costs.

Are prescription drugs covered?

Yes. All SNP plans must provide Medicare prescription drug coverage.

Do I need to choose a primary care doctor?

Generally, yes.

Do I have to get a referral to see a specialist?

In most cases, yes. Certain services, like yearly screening mammograms, don't require a referral.

What else do I need to know about this type of plan?

- These groups are eligible to enroll in a SNP:
  1. People who live in certain institutions (like nursing homes) or who require nursing care at home (also called an Institutional SNP or I-SNP).
  2. People who are eligible for both Medicare and Medicaid (also called a Dual Eligible SNP or D-SNP).
  3. People who have specific severe or disabling chronic conditions (like diabetes, End-Stage Renal Disease, HIV/AIDS, chronic heart failure, or dementia) (also called a Chronic condition SNP or C-SNP). Plans may further limit membership.

- A SNP provides benefits targeted to its members' special needs, including care coordination services.
- Visit Medicare.gov/plan-compare to see if there are SNPs available in your area. For information on what a specific SNP covers, check directly with the plan.
- If you need more information than what's listed on this page, check with the plan.

When can I join, switch, or drop a Medicare Advantage Plan?

- When you first become eligible for Medicare, you can sign up during your Initial Enrollment Period. See page 17.
- If you have Part A coverage and you get Part B for the first time during the General Enrollment Period, you can also join a Medicare Advantage Plan at that time. Your coverage may not start until July 1. See page 18.
- Between October 15–December 7, anyone with Medicare can join, switch, or drop a Medicare Advantage Plan. Your coverage will begin on January 1, as long as the plan gets your request by December 7.

If you drop a Medigap policy to join a Medicare Advantage Plan, you might not be able to get it back. Rules vary by state and your situation. See page 72 for more information.

> Always review the materials your plan sends you (like the "Annual Notice of Change" and "Evidence of Coverage"), and make sure your plan will still meet your needs for the following year. You can also visit the Medicare Plan Finder at Medicare.gov/plan-compare to compare your current plan with other available options.

Can I make changes to my coverage after December 7?

Between January 1–March 31 each year, you can make these changes during the **Medicare Advantage Open Enrollment Period**:

- If you're in a Medicare Advantage Plan (with or without drug coverage), you can switch to another Medicare Advantage Plan (with or without drug coverage).
- You can drop your Medicare Advantage Plan and return to Original Medicare. You'll also be able to join a Medicare Prescription Drug Plan.

During this period, you **can't**:

- Switch from Original Medicare to a Medicare Advantage Plan.
- Join a Medicare Prescription Drug Plan if you're in Original Medicare.
- Switch from one Medicare Prescription Drug Plan to another if you're in Original Medicare.

You can only make one change during this period, and any changes you make will be effective the first of the month after the plan gets your request. If you're returning to Original Medicare and joining a drug plan, you don't need to contact your Medicare Advantage Plan to disenroll. The disenrollment will happen automatically when you join the drug plan.

Note: If you enrolled in a Medicare Advantage Plan during your Initial Enrollment Period, you can change to another Medicare Advantage Plan (with or without drug coverage) or go back to Original Medicare (with or without a drug plan) within the first 3 months you have Medicare.

Important! ▷ **Thinking about joining a Medicare Advantage Plan between October 15–December 7, but aren't sure?** The Medicare Advantage Open Enrollment Period (January 1–March 31) gives you an opportunity to switch back to Original Medicare or change to a different Medicare Advantage Plan depending on which coverage works better for you.

Special Enrollment Periods

In most cases, you must stay enrolled for the calendar year starting the date your coverage begins. However, in certain situations, you may be able to join, switch, or drop a Medicare Advantage Plan during a Special Enrollment Period when certain events happen in your life. Check with your plan for more information.

How do I switch?

Follow these steps if you're already in a Medicare Advantage Plan and want to switch:

- **To switch to a new Medicare Advantage Plan,** simply join the plan you choose during one of the enrollment periods explained on page 65. You'll be disenrolled automatically from your old plan when your new plan's coverage begins.

- **To switch to Original Medicare,** contact your current plan, or call 1-800-MEDICARE (1-800-633-4227). TTY users can call 1-877-486-2048. If you don't have drug coverage, you should consider joining a Medicare Prescription Drug Plan to avoid paying a penalty if you decide to join later. You may also want to consider joining a Medicare Supplement Insurance (Medigap) policy if you're eligible. See page 69 for more information about buying a Medigap policy.

To join or switch Medicare Advantage Plans, visit Medicare.gov/plan-compare or call 1-800-MEDICARE.

For more details about Medicare Advantage Plans, visit Medicare.gov/publications to view the booklet "Understanding Medicare Advantage Plans."

Are there other types of Medicare health plans and projects?

Yes, some of these plans provide Medicare Part A (Hospital Insurance) and Medicare Part B (Medical Insurance) coverage, while others provide only Part B coverage. In addition, some also provide Part D prescription drug coverage. These plans have some of the same rules as Medicare Advantage Plans. However, each type of plan has special rules and exceptions, so you should contact any plans you're interested in to get more details.

Medicare Cost Plans

Medicare Cost Plans are a type of Medicare health plan available in certain, limited areas of the country. Here's what you should know about Medicare Cost Plans:

- You can join even if you only have Part B.
- If you have Part A and Part B and go to a non-network provider, the services are covered under Original Medicare. You'll pay the Part A and Part B coinsurance and deductibles.
- You can join anytime the Cost Plan is accepting new members.
- You can leave anytime and return to Original Medicare.
- You can either get your Medicare prescription drug coverage from the Cost Plan (if offered) or you can join a Medicare Prescription Drug Plan. Even if the Cost Plan offers prescription drug coverage, you can choose to get drug coverage from a separate Medicare drug plan.

  Note: You can add or drop Medicare prescription drug coverage only at certain times. See pages 74–75.

For more information about Medicare Cost Plans, visit the Medicare Plan Finder at **Medicare.gov/plan-compare**. Your State Health Insurance Assistance Program (SHIP) can also give you more information. See pages 109–112 for the phone number.

Programs of All-inclusive Care for the Elderly (PACE)

PACE is a Medicare and Medicaid program offered in many states that allows people who otherwise need a nursing home-level of care to remain in the community. To qualify for PACE, you must meet these conditions:

- You're 55 or older.
- You live in the service area of a PACE organization.
- You're certified by your state as needing a nursing home-level of care.
- At the time you join, you're able to live safely in the community with the help of PACE services.

PACE covers all Medicare- and Medicaid-covered care and services, and other services that the PACE team of health care professionals decides are necessary to improve and maintain your health. This includes prescription drugs, as well as any other medically necessary care, like doctor or health care provider visits, transportation, home care, hospital visits, and even nursing home stays when necessary.

If you have Medicaid, you won't have to pay a monthly premium for the long-term care portion of the PACE benefit. If you have Medicare but not Medicaid, you'll be charged a monthly premium to cover the long-term care portion of the PACE benefit and a premium for Medicare Part D drugs. However, in PACE, there's never a deductible or copayment for any drug, service, or care approved by the PACE team of health care professionals.

Visit **Medicare.gov/plan-compare** to see if there's a PACE organization that serves your community.

Medicare Innovation Projects

Medicare develops innovative models, demonstrations, and pilot projects to test and measure the effect of potential changes in Medicare. These projects help to find new ways to improve health care quality and reduce costs. Usually, they operate only a limited time for a specific group of people and/or are offered only in specific areas. Examples of current models, demonstrations, and pilot projects include innovations in primary care, care related to specific procedures (like hip and knee replacements), cancer care, and care for people with End-Stage Renal Disease (ESRD). To learn more about the current Medicare models, demonstrations, and pilot projects, call 1-800-MEDICARE (1-800-633-4227). TTY users can call 1-877-486-2048.

Medicare Supplement Insurance (Medigap) policies

Original Medicare pays for much, but not all, of the cost for covered health care services and supplies. Medicare Supplement Insurance policies, sold by private companies, can help pay some of the remaining health care costs for covered services and supplies, like copayments, coinsurance, and deductibles. **Medicare Supplement Insurance policies are also called Medigap policies.**

Some Medigap policies also offer coverage for services that Original Medicare doesn't cover, like medical care when you travel outside the U.S. Generally, Medigap policies don't cover long-term care (like care in a nursing home), vision or dental care, hearing aids, eyeglasses, or private-duty nursing.

Medigap policies are standardized

Every Medigap policy must follow federal and state laws designed to protect you, and they must be clearly identified as "Medicare Supplement Insurance." Insurance companies can sell you only a "standardized" policy identified in most states by letters A through D, F, G, and K through N. All policies offer the same basic benefits, but some offer additional benefits so you can choose which one meets your needs. In Massachusetts, Minnesota, and Wisconsin, Medigap policies are standardized in a different way.

Important! Starting January 1, 2020, Medigap plans sold to people who are new to Medicare won't be allowed to cover the Part B deductible. Because of this, Plans C and F won't be available to people who are newly eligible for Medicare on or after January 1, 2020. If you already have either of these 2 plans (or the high deductible version of Plan F) or are covered by one of these plans before January 1, 2020, you'll be able to keep your plan. If you were eligible for Medicare before January 1, 2020, but not yet enrolled, you may be able to buy one of these plans.

⭐ **Note:** Definitions of blue words are on pages 113–116.

How do I compare Medigap policies?

The chart below shows basic information about the different benefits that Medigap policies cover for 2020. If a percentage appears, the Medigap plan covers that percentage of the benefit, and you're responsible for the rest.

Benefits	Medicare Supplement Insurance (Medigap) plans									
	A	B	C	D	F*	G	K	L	M	N
Medicare Part A coinsurance and hospital costs (up to an additional 365 days after Medicare benefits are used)	100%	100%	100%	100%	100%	100%	100%	100%	100%	100%
Medicare Part B coinsurance or copayment	100%	100%	100%	100%	100%	100%	50%	75%	100%	100%***
Blood (first 3 pints)	100%	100%	100%	100%	100%	100%	50%	75%	100%	100%
Part A hospice care coinsurance or copayment	100%	100%	100%	100%	100%	100%	50%	75%	100%	100%
Skilled nursing facility care coinsurance			100%	100%	100%	100%	50%	75%	100%	100%
Part A deductible		100%	100%	100%	100%	100%	50%	75%	50%	100%
Part B deductible			100%		100%					
Part B excess charges					100%	100%				
Foreign travel emergency (up to plan limits)			80%	80%	80%	80%			80%	80%
							Out-of-pocket limit in 2020**			
							$5,880	$2,940		

* Plan F also offers a high-deductible plan in some states. With this option, you must pay for Medicare-covered costs (coinsurance, copayments, and deductibles) up to the deductible amount of $2,340 in 2020 before your policy pays anything. (Plans C and F won't be available to people who are newly eligible for Medicare on or after January 1, 2020. See previous page for more information.)

** For Plans K and L, after you meet your out-of-pocket yearly limit and your yearly Part B deductible ($198 in 2020), the Medigap plan pays 100% of covered services for the rest of the calendar year.

*** Plan N pays 100% of the Part B coinsurance, except for a copayment of up to $20 for some office visits and up to a $50 copayment for emergency room visits that don't result in an inpatient admission.

What else should I know about Medicare Supplement Insurance (Medigap)?

Important facts

- You must have Part A and Part B.
- You pay the private insurance company a monthly premium for your Medigap policy in addition to your monthly Part B premium that you pay to Medicare. Also, if you join a Medigap policy and a Medicare Prescription Drug Plan offered by the same company, you may need to make 2 separate premium payments for your coverage. Contact the company to find out how to pay your premiums.
- A Medigap policy only covers one person. Spouses must buy separate policies.
- You can't have prescription drug coverage in both your Medigap policy and a Medicare drug plan. See page 81. However, the same insurance company may offer Medigap policies and Medicare Prescription Drug Plans.
- It's important to compare Medigap policies since the costs can vary between insurance companies for exactly the same coverage, and may go up as you get older. Some states limit Medigap premium costs.
- In some states, you may be able to buy another type of Medigap policy called Medicare SELECT. If you buy a Medicare SELECT policy, you have rights to change your mind within 12 months and switch to a standard Medigap policy.

When to buy

- The best time to buy a Medigap policy is during your Medigap Open Enrollment Period. This 6-month period begins on the first day of the month in which you're 65 or older **and** enrolled in Part B. (Some states have additional Open Enrollment Periods.) **After this enrollment period, you may not be able to buy a Medigap policy. If you're able to buy one, it may cost more.**
- If you delay enrolling in Part B because you have group health coverage based on your (or your spouse's) current employment, your Medigap Open Enrollment Period won't start until you sign up for Part B.
- Federal law generally doesn't require insurance companies to sell Medigap policies to people under 65. If you're under 65, you might not be able to buy the Medigap policy you want, or any Medigap policy, until you turn 65. However, some states require Medigap insurance companies to sell Medigap policies to people under 65. If you're able to buy one, it may cost more.

Can I have a Medigap policy and a Medicare Advantage Plan?

- If you have a Medicare Advantage Plan, it's illegal for anyone to sell you a Medigap policy unless you're switching back to Original Medicare. If you're not planning to leave your Medicare Advantage Plan, and someone tries to sell you a Medigap policy, report it to your State Insurance Department.

- If you have a Medigap policy and join a Medicare Advantage Plan, you may want to drop your Medigap policy. Your Medigap policy **can't** be used to pay your Medicare Advantage Plan copayments, deductibles, and premiums. If you want to cancel your Medigap policy, contact your insurance company. In most cases, if you drop your Medigap policy to join a Medicare Advantage Plan, you won't be able to get it back.

- If you join a Medicare Advantage Plan for the first time, and you aren't happy with the plan, you'll have special rights under federal law to buy a Medigap policy and a Medicare Prescription Drug Plan if you return to Original Medicare within 12 months of joining the Medicare Advantage Plan.

  - If you had a Medigap policy before you joined, you may be able to get the same policy back if the company still sells it. If it isn't available, you can buy another Medigap policy.

  - If you joined a Medicare Advantage Plan when you were first eligible for Medicare, you can choose from any Medigap policy within the first year of joining.

  - Some states provide additional special rights to buy a Medigap policy.

Where can I get more information?

- Visit Medicare.gov to find policies in your area.
- Visit Medicare.gov/publications to view the booklet "Choosing a Medigap Policy: A Guide to Health Insurance for People with Medicare."
- Call your State Insurance Department. Visit Medicare.gov/contacts, or call 1-800-MEDICARE (1-800-633-4227) to get the phone number. TTY users can call 1-877-486-2048.
- Call your State Health Insurance Assistance Program (SHIP). See pages 109–112 for the phone number.

Medicare prescription drug coverage (Part D)

How does Medicare prescription drug coverage (Part D) work?

Medicare prescription drug coverage is an optional benefit. Medicare drug coverage is offered to everyone with Medicare. Even if you don't use prescription drugs now, you should consider joining a Medicare drug plan. If you decide not to join a Medicare drug plan when you're first eligible, and you don't have other creditable prescription drug coverage or get Extra Help, you'll likely pay a late enrollment penalty if you join a plan later. Generally, you'll pay this penalty for as long as you have Medicare prescription drug coverage. See pages 77–78. To get Medicare prescription drug coverage, you must join a plan approved by Medicare that offers Medicare drug coverage. Each plan can vary in cost and specific drugs covered. Visit Medicare.gov/plan-compare for more information about plans in your area.

There are 2 ways to get Medicare prescription drug coverage:

1. **Medicare Prescription Drug Plans.** These plans (sometimes called "PDPs") add drug coverage to Original Medicare, some Medicare Cost Plans, some Medicare Private Fee-for-Service (PFFS) plans, and Medicare Medical Savings Account (MSA) plans. You must have Part A and/or Part B to join a Medicare Prescription Drug Plan.

2. **Medicare Advantage Plans or other Medicare health plans that offer Medicare prescription drug coverage.** You get all of your Part A, Part B, and prescription drug coverage (Part D), through these plans. Medicare Advantage Plans with prescription drug coverage are sometimes called "MA-PDs." Remember, you must have Part A and Part B to join a Medicare Advantage Plan, and not all of these plans offer drug coverage.

In either case, you must live in the service area of the Medicare drug plan you want to join. **Both types of plans are called "Medicare drug plans" in this handbook.**

⭐ **Note:** Definitions of blue words are on pages 113–116.

Important!

If you have employer or union coverage
Call your benefits administrator before you make any changes, or sign up for any other coverage. Signing up for other coverage could cause you to lose your employer or union health and drug coverage for you and your dependents. If you lose your employer or union coverage, you may not be able to get it back. If you want to know how Medicare prescription drug coverage works with other drug coverage you may have, see page 58.

When can I join, switch, or drop a Medicare drug plan?

- When you first become eligible for Medicare, you can join during your Initial Enrollment Period. See page 17.
- If you get Part A and Part B for the first time during the General Enrollment Period, you can also join a Medicare drug plan from April 1– June 30. Your coverage will start on July 1.
- You can join, switch, or drop a Medicare drug plan between October 15– December 7 each year. Your changes will take effect on January 1 of the following year, as long as the plan gets your request before December 7.
- If you're enrolled in a Medicare Advantage Plan, you can join, switch, or drop a plan during the Medicare Advantage Open Enrollment Period, between January 1–March 31 each year. See page 65 for more information.
- If you qualify for a Special Enrollment Period. See below.

Special Enrollment Periods
Special Enrollment Periods are times when you can join, switch, or drop your Medicare drug coverage if you meet certain requirements. Generally you must stay enrolled in your Medicare drug plan for the entire year, but you may be able to change your coverage mid-year if you qualify for a Special Enrollment Period when certain events happen in your life. Check with your plan for more information.

How do I switch?
You can switch to a new Medicare drug plan simply by joining another drug plan during one of the times listed above. **You don't need to cancel your old Medicare drug plan.** Your old Medicare drug plan coverage will end when your new drug plan coverage begins. You should get a letter from your new Medicare drug plan telling you when your coverage with the new plan begins. You can switch plans by calling 1-800-MEDICARE (1-800-633-4227). TTY users can call 1-877-486-2048.

How do I drop a Medicare drug plan?
If you want to drop your Medicare drug plan and don't want to join a new plan, you can only do so during certain times. See page 74. You can disenroll by calling 1-800-MEDICARE. You can also send a letter to the plan to tell them you want to disenroll. If you drop your plan and want to join another Medicare drug plan later, you have to wait for an enrollment period. You may have to pay a late enrollment penalty if you don't have creditable prescription drug coverage. See pages 77–78.

Read the information you get from your plan
Review the "Evidence of Coverage" (EOC) and "Annual Notice of Change" (ANOC) your plan sends you each year. The EOC gives you details about what the plan covers, how much you pay, and more. The ANOC includes any changes in coverage, costs, provider networks, service area, and more that will be effective in January. If you don't get these important documents in early fall, contact your plan.

How much do I pay?
Below and continued on the next page are descriptions of what you pay in your Medicare drug plan. **Your actual drug plan costs will vary depending on:**

- Your prescriptions and whether they're on your plan's formulary (list of covered drugs) and depending on what "tier" the drug is in. See page 79.
- Which phase of your drug benefit that you're in (some examples include whether or not you met your deductible, if you're in the catastrophic coverage phase, etc.)
- The plan you choose. Remember, plan coverage and costs can change each year.
- Which pharmacy you use (whether it offers preferred or standard cost sharing, is out-of-network, or is mail order). Your out-of-pocket prescription drug costs may be less at a preferred pharmacy because it has agreed with your plan to charge less.
- Whether you get Extra Help paying your Part D costs. See pages 83–85.

> You may be able to lower the cost of your prescriptions. Some ways include choosing generics over brand name or paying the non-insurance cost of a drug. Ask your pharmacist—they can tell you if there's a less expensive option available. You can also submit your receipts to your plan to have these costs counted toward your yearly out-of-pocket costs. Check with your plan to find out how.

Monthly premium

Most drug plans charge a monthly fee that varies by plan. You pay this in addition to the Part B premium. If you're in a Medicare Advantage Plan or a Medicare Cost Plan that includes Medicare prescription drug coverage, the monthly premium may include an amount for prescription drug coverage.

Note: Contact your drug plan (not Social Security or the Railroad Retirement Board (RRB)) if you want your premium deducted from your monthly Social Security or RRB payment. If you want to stop premium deductions and get billed directly, contact your drug plan.

Important! ▸ **If you have a higher income, you might pay more for your Part D coverage.** If your income is above a certain limit ($87,000 if you file individually or $174,000 if you're married and file jointly), you'll pay an extra amount in addition to your plan premium (sometimes called "Part D-IRMAA"). You'll also have to pay this extra amount if you're in a Medicare Advantage Plan that includes drug coverage. This doesn't affect everyone, so most people won't have to pay a higher amount. If you have to pay a higher amount for Part D, you'll also pay an extra amount for your Part B premium. See page 22.

Usually, the extra amount will be deducted from your Social Security check. If you get benefits from the Railroad Retirement Board (RRB), the extra amount will be deducted from your RRB check. **If you're billed the amount by Medicare or the RRB, you must pay the extra amount to Medicare or the RRB and not your plan.** If you don't pay the extra amount, you could lose your Part D coverage. You may not be able to enroll in another plan right away, and you may have to pay a late enrollment penalty for as long as you have Part D.

If you have to pay an extra amount and you disagree (for example, you have a life event that lowers your income), visit socialsecurity.gov or call Social Security at 1-800-772-1213. TTY users can call 1-800-325-0778.

Yearly deductible

This is the amount you must pay before your drug plan begins to pay its share of your covered drugs. Some drug plans don't have a deductible.

Copayments or coinsurance

These are the amounts you pay for your covered prescriptions after the deductible (if the plan has one). You pay your share and your drug plan pays its share for covered drugs. If you pay coinsurance, these amounts may vary throughout the year due to changes in the drug's total cost.

Catastrophic coverage

Once you've met your plan's out-of-pocket cost requirements for the year, you automatically get "catastrophic coverage." With catastrophic coverage, you only pay a reduced coinsurance amount or copayment for covered drugs for the rest of the year.

Note: If you get Extra Help, you won't have some of these costs. See pages 83–84.

Important! Visit Medicare.gov/plan-compare to get specific Medicare drug plan costs, and call the plans you're interested in to get more details. For help comparing plan costs, contact your State Health Insurance Assistance Program (SHIP). See pages 109–112 for the phone number.

What's the Part D late enrollment penalty?

The late enrollment penalty is an amount that's permanently added to your Part D premium. You may owe a late enrollment penalty if at any time after your Initial Enrollment Period is over, there's a period of 63 or more days in a row when you don't have Part D or other creditable prescription drug coverage. You'll generally have to pay the penalty for as long as you have Part D coverage.

Note: If you get Extra Help, you don't pay a late enrollment penalty.

3 ways to avoid paying a penalty:

1. **Join a Medicare drug plan when you're first eligible.** Even if you don't take prescriptions now, you should consider joining a Medicare Prescription Drug Plan or a Medicare Advantage Plan that offers drug coverage to avoid a penalty. You may be able to find a plan that meets your needs with little to no monthly premiums. See pages 5–9 to learn more about your choices.

2. **Enroll in a Medicare drug plan if you lose other creditable coverage.** Creditable prescription drug coverage could include drug coverage from a current or former employer or union, TRICARE, Indian Health Service, the Department of Veterans Affairs, or individual health insurance coverage. Your plan must tell you each year if your drug coverage is creditable coverage. If you go 63 days or more in a row without a Medicare drug plan or other creditable prescription drug coverage, you may have to pay a penalty if you join later.

3. **Keep records showing when you had creditable drug coverage, and tell your plan if they ask about it.** If you don't tell the plan about your creditable prescription drug coverage, you may have to pay a penalty for as long as you have Part D coverage.

How much more will I pay?

The cost of the late enrollment penalty depends on how long you didn't have creditable prescription drug coverage. Currently, the late enrollment penalty is calculated by multiplying 1% of the "national base beneficiary premium" ($32.74 in 2020) by the number of full, uncovered months that you were eligible but didn't join a Medicare drug plan and went without other creditable prescription drug coverage. The final amount is rounded to the nearest $.10 and added to your monthly premium. Since the "national base beneficiary premium" may increase each year, the penalty amount may also increase each year. After you join a Medicare drug plan, the plan will tell you if you owe a penalty and what your premium will be.

Example:

Mrs. Martin didn't join a drug plan when she was first eligible—by June 2017. She doesn't have prescription drug coverage from any other source. She joined a Medicare drug plan during November 2019, and her coverage began on January 1, 2020.

Since Mrs. Martin was without creditable prescription drug coverage from July 2017–December 2019, her penalty in 2020 is 30% (1% for each of the 30 months) of $32.74 (the national base beneficiary premium for 2020), which is $9.82. The final amount is rounded to the nearest $.10, so she'll be charged $9.80 each month in addition to her plan's monthly premium in 2020. She'll continue to pay a penalty for as long as she has Part D coverage, and the amount may go up each year.

Here's the math:

.30 (30% penalty) × **$32.74** (2020 base beneficiary premium) = **$9.82**

$9.80 = Mrs. Martin's monthly late enrollment penalty for 2020 (rounded to the nearest $.10)

What if I don't agree with the penalty?

If you disagree with your penalty, you can ask for a review or reconsideration. Generally, you must request this review within 60 days from the date on the first letter you get stating you have to pay a late enrollment penalty. You'll need to fill out a reconsideration request form (that your Medicare drug plan will send you) by the date listed in the letter. You can provide proof that supports your case, like information about previous creditable prescription drug coverage. If you need help, call your plan.

Which drugs are covered?

Information about a plan's list of covered drugs (called a "formulary") isn't included in this handbook because each plan has its own formulary. Many Medicare drug plans place drugs into different "tiers" on their formularies. Drugs in each tier have a different cost. Drugs in a lower tier will generally cost less than a drug in a higher tier. In some cases, if your drug is in a higher tier and your prescriber thinks you need that drug instead of a similar drug in a lower tier, you or your prescriber can ask your plan for an exception. See page 92 for more information on exceptions.

Formularies can be changed by the plan. Your plan will notify you of any formulary changes that affect drugs you're taking.

Contact the plan for its current formulary, or visit the plan's website. You can also visit the Medicare Plan Finder at Medicare.gov/plan-compare, or call 1-800-MEDICARE (1-800-633-4227). TTY users can call 1-877-486-2048. Your plan will notify you of any formulary changes.

Important! Each month that you fill a prescription, your drug plan mails you an "Explanation of Benefits" (EOB) notice. Review your notice and check it for mistakes. Contact your plan if you have questions or find mistakes. If you suspect fraud, call the Medicare Drug Integrity Contractor (MEDIC) at 1-877-7SAFERX (1-877-772-3379). See page 98 for more information.

Plans may have these coverage rules for certain drugs:

- **Prior authorization:** You and/or your prescriber must contact the drug plan before you can fill certain prescriptions. Your prescriber may need to show that the drug is medically necessary for the plan to cover it.

  Plans may also use prior authorization when they cover a medication for certain medical conditions, but not all medical conditions for which a drug is approved. When this occurs, plans will likely have alternative medications on their formulary (drug list) for the other medical conditions, for which the drug can be prescribed.

- **Quantity limits:** Limits on how much medication you can get at a time.

- **Step therapy:** In most cases, you must try one or more similar, lower-cost drugs before the plan will cover the prescribed drug.

- **Prescription safety checks at the pharmacy (including opioid pain medications):** Before your prescriptions are filled, your Medicare drug plan and pharmacy perform additional safety checks, like checking for drug interactions and incorrect dosages. These checks also include checking for possible unsafe amounts of opioids, limiting the days supply of a first prescription for opioids, and use of opioids at the same time as benzodiazepines (commonly used for anxiety and sleep). Opioid pain medications (like oxycodone and hydrocodone) can help with certain types of pain, but have serious risks like addiction, overdose, and death. These risks are increased when opioids are taken with certain other medications.

- **Drug Management Programs:** Some Medicare drug plans have a program in place to help you use these opioids and benzodiazepines safely. If you get opioids from multiple doctors or pharmacies, your plan will contact the doctors who prescribed these drugs to make sure they are medically necessary and that you're using them appropriately.

If your Medicare drug plan decides your use of prescription opioids and benzodiazepines may not be safe, the plan will send you a letter in advance. This letter will tell you if the plan will limit coverage of these drugs for you, or if you'll be required to get the prescriptions for these drugs only from a doctor or pharmacy that you select. You and your doctor have the right to appeal these limitations if you disagree with the plan's decision (see page 90). The letter will also tell you how to contact the plan if you have questions or would like to make an appeal.

The opioid safety reviews at the pharmacy and the Drug Management Programs generally don't apply to you if you have cancer, getting palliative or end-of-life care, are in hospice, or reside in a long-term care facility.

If you or your prescriber believe that one of these coverage rules should be waived, you can ask for an exception. See page 92.

If you're prescribed opioids:

- Talk with your doctor about your dosage and the length of time you'll be taking them. You and your doctor may decide later you don't need to take all of your prescription.
- Talk with your doctor about other options that Medicare covers to treat your pain, like non-opioid medications and devices, physical therapy, individual and group therapy, behavioral health integration services, and more. There also may be other pain treatment options available that Medicare doesn't cover.
- Never take opioids in greater amounts or more often than prescribed.
- Safely dispose of unused prescription opioids through your community drug take-back program or your pharmacy mail-back program.

For more information on safe and effective pain management and opioid use, visit Medicare.gov or call 1-800-MEDICARE (1-800-633-4227). TTY users can call 1-877-486-2048.

Do you get automatic prescription refills in the mail?

Some people with Medicare get their prescription drugs by using an "automatic refill" service that automatically delivers prescription drugs when they're about to run out. To make sure you still need a prescription before they send you a refill, prescription drug plans may offer a voluntary auto-ship program. Contact your plan for more information.

Medication Therapy Management (MTM) Program

Plans with Medicare prescription drug coverage must offer additional Medication Therapy Management (MTM) services to plan members who meet certain requirements. Members who qualify can get these MTM services to help them understand how to manage their medications and use them safely. The MTM services offered may vary in some plans. MTM services are free and usually include a discussion with a pharmacist or health care provider to review your medications.

The pharmacist or health care provider may talk with you about:

- How well your medications are working
- Whether your medications have side effects
- If there might be interactions between the drugs you're taking
- Whether your costs can be lowered
- Other problems you're having

Visit **Medicare.gov/plan-compare** to get general information about program eligibility for your Medicare drug plan or for other plans that interest you. Contact each drug plan for specific details.

How do other insurance and programs work with Part D?

Medicaid: If you have Medicare and full Medicaid coverage, Medicare covers your Part D prescription drugs. Medicaid may still cover some drugs that Medicare doesn't cover.

Employer or union health coverage: This is health coverage from your, your spouse's, or other family member's current or former employer or union. If you have prescription drug coverage based on your current or previous employment, your employer or union will notify you each year to let you know if your prescription drug coverage is creditable. **Keep the information you get.** Call your benefits administrator for more information before making any changes to your coverage.

Note: If you join a Medicare drug plan, you, your spouse, or your dependents may lose your employer or union health coverage.

COBRA: This is a federal law that may allow you to temporarily keep employer or union health coverage after the employment ends or after you lose coverage as a dependent of the covered employee. As explained on page 18, there may be reasons why you should take Part B instead of, or in addition to, COBRA coverage. However, if you take COBRA and it includes creditable prescription drug coverage, you'll have a Special Enrollment Period to join a Medicare drug plan without paying a penalty when the COBRA coverage ends. Talk with your State Health Insurance Assistance Program (SHIP) to see if COBRA is a good choice for you. See pages 109–112 for the phone number.

Medicare Supplement Insurance (Medigap) policy with prescription drug coverage: You may choose to join a Medicare drug plan because most Medigap drug coverage isn't creditable, and you may pay more if you join a drug plan later. See pages 77–78. Medigap policies can no longer be sold with prescription drug coverage, but if you have drug coverage under a current Medigap policy, you can keep it. If you join a Medicare Prescription Drug Plan, tell your Medigap insurance company so they can remove the prescription drug coverage under your Medigap policy and adjust your premiums. Call your Medigap insurance company for more information.

Note: Keep any creditable prescription drug coverage information you get from your plan. You may need it if you decide to join a Medicare drug plan later. Don't send creditable coverage letters or certificates to Medicare.

How does other government insurance work with Part D?

The types of insurance listed below are all considered creditable prescription drug coverage, and in most cases, it will be to your advantage to keep this coverage if you have it.

Federal Employee Health Benefits (FEHB) Program: This is health coverage for current and retired federal employees and covered family members. FEHB plans usually include prescription drug coverage, so you don't need to join a Medicare drug plan. However, if you decide to join a Medicare drug plan, you can keep your FEHB plan, and in most cases, the Medicare plan will pay first. For more information, visit opm.gov/healthcare-insurance/healthcare, or call the Office of Personnel Management at 1-888-767-6738. TTY users can call 1-800-878-5707. If you're an active federal employee, contact your Benefits Officer. Visit apps.opm.gov/abo for a list of Benefits Officers. You can also call your plan if you have questions.

Veterans' benefits: This is health coverage for veterans and people who have served in the U.S. military. You may be able to get prescription drug coverage through the U.S. Department of Veterans Affairs (VA) program. You may join a Medicare Prescription Drug Plan, but if you do, you can't use both types of coverage for the same prescription at the same time. For more information, visit va.gov, or call the VA at 1-800-827-1000. TTY users can call 1-800-829-4833.

TRICARE (military health benefits): This is a health care plan for active-duty service members, military retirees, and their families. **Most people with TRICARE who are entitled to Part A must have Part B to keep TRICARE prescription drug benefits.** If you have TRICARE, you don't need to join a Medicare Prescription Drug Plan. However, if you do, your Medicare Prescription Drug Plan pays first, and TRICARE pays second.

If you join a Medicare Advantage Plan with prescription drug coverage, your Medicare Advantage Plan and TRICARE may coordinate their benefits if your Medicare Advantage Plan network pharmacy is also a TRICARE network pharmacy. Otherwise, you can file your own claim to get paid back for your out-of-pocket expenses. For more information, visit tricare.mil, or call the TRICARE Pharmacy Program at 1-877-363-1303. TTY users can call 1-877-540-6261.

Indian Health Service (IHS): The IHS is the primary health care provider to the American Indian/Alaska Native Medicare population. The Indian health care system, consisting of tribal, urban, and federally operated IHS health programs, delivers a spectrum of clinical and preventive health services through a network of hospitals, clinics, and other entities. Many Indian health facilities participate in the Medicare prescription drug program. If you get prescription drugs through an Indian health facility, you'll continue to get drugs at no cost to you, and your coverage won't be interrupted. Joining a Medicare drug plan may help your Indian health facility because the drug plan pays the Indian health facility for the cost of your prescriptions. Talk to your local Indian health benefits coordinator who can help you choose a plan that meets your needs and tell you how Medicare works with the Indian health care system.

Note: If you're getting care through an IHS or tribal health facility or program without being charged, you can continue to do so for some or all of your care. Getting Medicare doesn't affect your ability to get services through the IHS and tribal health facilities.

SECTION 7

Get help paying your health & prescription drug costs

What if I need help paying my Medicare prescription drug costs?

If you have limited income and resources, you may qualify for help to pay for some health care and prescription drug costs.

Extra Help is a Medicare program to help people with limited income and resources pay Medicare prescription drug costs. You may qualify for Extra Help if your yearly income and resources are below these limits in 2019:

	Yearly income	Other resources
Single person	less than $18,735 per year	less than $14,390 per year
Married person living with a spouse and no other dependents	less than $25,365	less than $28,720 per year

These amounts may change in 2020. You may qualify even if you have a higher income (like if you still work, live in Alaska or Hawaii, or have dependents living with you). Resources include money in a checking or savings account, stocks, bonds, mutual funds, and Individual Retirement Accounts (IRAs). Resources **don't** include your home, car, household items, burial plot, up to $1,500 for burial expenses (per person), or life insurance policies.

If you qualify for Extra Help and join a Medicare drug plan, you'll:

- Get help paying your Medicare drug plan's costs.
- Have no late enrollment penalty.

Note: Extra Help isn't available in Puerto Rico, the U.S. Virgin Islands, Guam, the Northern Mariana Islands, or American Samoa. See page 88 for information about programs that are available in those areas.

⭐ **Note:** Definitions of blue words are on pages 113–116.

Most people with Medicare can only make changes to their drug coverage certain times of the year. If you newly get, lose, or have a change in your Medicaid or Extra Help status, you may get a Special Enrollment Period to change drug plans. Check with your plan for more information.

You automatically qualify for Extra Help if you have Medicare and meet any of these conditions:

- You have full Medicaid coverage.
- You get help from your state Medicaid program paying your Part B premiums (in a Medicare Savings Program). See pages 86–87.
- You get Supplemental Security Income (SSI) benefits.

To let you know you automatically qualify for Extra Help, Medicare will mail you a purple letter that you should keep for your records. You don't need to apply for Extra Help if you get this letter.

- If you aren't already in a Medicare drug plan, you must join one to use this Extra Help.
- If you're not enrolled in a Medicare drug plan, Medicare may enroll you in one so that you'll be able to use the Extra Help. If Medicare enrolls you in a plan, you'll get a yellow or green letter letting you know when your coverage begins, and you'll have a Special Enrollment Period to change plans.
- Different plans cover different drugs. Check to see if the plan you're enrolled in covers the drugs you use and if you can go to the pharmacies you want. Visit **Medicare.gov/plan-compare**, or call 1-800-MEDICARE (1-800-633-4227) to compare it with other plans in your area. TTY users can call 1-877-486-2048.
- If you have Medicaid and live in certain institutions (like a nursing home) or get home- and community-based services, you pay nothing for your covered prescription drugs.

If you don't want to join a Medicare drug plan (for example, because you want only your employer or union coverage), call the plan listed in your letter, or call 1-800-MEDICARE (1-800-633-4227). TTY users can call 1-877-486-2048. Tell them you don't want to be in a Medicare drug plan (you want to "opt out"). If you continue to qualify for Extra Help or if your employer or union coverage is creditable prescription drug coverage, you won't have to pay a penalty if you join later.

Important! If you have employer or union coverage and you join a Medicare drug plan, you may lose your employer or union coverage (for you and your dependents) even if you qualify for Extra Help. Call your employer's benefits administrator before you join a Medicare drug plan.

Drug costs in 2020 for people who qualify will be no more than $3.60 for each generic drug and $8.95 for each brand-name drug. Look on the Extra Help letters you get, or contact your plan to find out your exact costs.

If you didn't automatically qualify for Extra Help, you can apply anytime:
- Visit socialsecurity.gov/i1020 to apply online.
- Call Social Security at 1-800-772-1213. TTY users can call 1-800-325-0778.

Note: When you apply for Extra Help, you also can start your application process for the Medicare Savings Programs. These state programs provide help with other Medicare costs. Social Security will send information to your state unless you tell them not to on the Extra Help application.

To get answers to your questions about Extra Help and help choosing a drug plan, call your State Health Insurance Assistance Program (SHIP). See pages 109–112 for the phone number. You can also call 1-800-MEDICARE.

What if I need help paying my Medicare health care costs?

Medicare Savings Programs
If you have limited income and resources, you may be able to get help from your state to pay your Medicare costs if you meet certain conditions.

There are 4 kinds of Medicare Savings Programs:
1. **Qualified Medicare Beneficiary (QMB) Program:** If you're eligible, the QMB Program helps pay for Part A and/or Part B premiums. In addition, Medicare providers aren't allowed to bill you for services and items Medicare covers, including deductibles, coinsurance, and copayments (except outpatient prescription drugs). If you get a bill for these charges, tell your provider or debt collector that you're in the QMB Program and can't be charged for items and services Medicare covers, including deductibles, coinsurance, and copayments. If you've already made payments on a bill for services and items Medicare covers, you have the right to a refund.

    Note: To make sure your provider knows you're in the QMB Program, show both your Medicare and Medicaid or QMB card each time you get care. You can also give your provider a copy of your "Medicare Summary Notice" (MSN). Your MSN will show you're in the QMB Program and shouldn't be billed. Log in to your MyMedicare.gov account at any time to view your MSN or sign up to get your MSNs electronically.

    If your provider won't stop billing you, call us at 1-800-MEDICARE (1-800-633-4227). TTY users can call 1-877-486-2048. We can confirm that you're in the QMB Program. We can also ask your provider to stop billing you, and refund any payments you've already made.

2. **Specified Low-Income Medicare Beneficiary (SLMB) Program:** Helps pay Part B premiums only.

3. **Qualifying Individual (QI) Program:** Helps pay Part B premiums only. Funding for QI benefits is limited, and the applications are granted on a first come, first-served basis.

4. **Qualified Disabled and Working Individuals (QDWI) Program:** Helps pay Part A premiums only. You may qualify for this program if you have a disability and are working.

> If you qualify for a QMB, SLMB, or QI Program, you automatically qualify to get Extra Help paying for Medicare prescription drug coverage. See pages 83–85.

Important! The names of these programs and how they work may vary by state. Medicare Savings Programs aren't available in Puerto Rico or the U.S. Virgin Islands.

How do I qualify?

In most cases, to qualify for a Medicare Savings Program, you must have income and resources below a certain limit.

States have different limits and ways of counting your income and resources, so you should check with your state Medicaid office to see if you qualify.

For more information

- Call or visit your Medicaid office (State Medical Assistance Office), and ask for information about Medicare Savings Programs. To get the phone number for your state, visit **Medicare.gov/contacts**. You can also call 1-800-MEDICARE (1-800-633-4227). TTY users can call 1-877-486-2048.
- Contact your State Health Insurance Assistance Program (SHIP). See pages 109–112 for the phone number.

Medicaid

Medicaid is a joint federal and state program that helps pay health care costs if you have limited income and resources and meet other requirements. Some people qualify for both Medicare and Medicaid.

What does Medicaid cover?

- If you have Medicare and full Medicaid coverage, most of your health care costs are covered. You can get your Medicare coverage through Original Medicare or a Medicare Advantage Plan.
- If you have Medicare and/or full Medicaid coverage, Medicare covers your Part D prescription drugs. Medicaid may still cover some drugs that Medicare doesn't cover.
- People with Medicaid may get coverage for services that Medicare doesn't cover or only partially covers, like nursing home care, personal care, transportation to medical services, home- and community-based services, and dental, vision, and hearing services.

How do I qualify?

- Medicaid programs vary from state to state. They may also have different names, like "Medical Assistance" or "Medi-Cal."
- Each state has different income and resource requirements.
- In most cases, you need to be enrolled in Medicare, if eligible, to get Medicaid.
- Call your Medicaid office for more information and to see if you qualify. Visit **Medicare.gov/contacts**, or call 1-800-MEDICARE.

Demonstration plans for people who have both Medicare and Medicaid

Medicare is working with some states and health plans to offer demonstration plans for certain people who have both Medicare and Medicaid, called Medicare-Medicaid Plans. If you're interested in joining a Medicare-Medicaid Plan, visit **Medicare.gov/plan-compare** to see if one is available in your area and if you qualify.

State Pharmacy Assistance Programs (SPAPs)

Many states have SPAPs that help certain people pay for prescription drugs based on financial need, age, or medical condition. To find out if there's an SPAP in your state and how it works, call your State Health Insurance Assistance Program (SHIP). See pages 109–112 for the phone number.

Pharmaceutical Assistance Programs (also called Patient Assistance Programs)

Many major drug manufacturers offer assistance programs for people with Medicare drug coverage who meet certain requirements. Visit Medicare.gov/pharmaceutical-assistance-program to learn more about Pharmaceutical Assistance Programs.

Programs of All-inclusive Care for the Elderly (PACE)

PACE is a Medicare and Medicaid program offered in many states that allows people who need a nursing home-level of care to remain in the community. See page 68 for more information.

Supplemental Security Income (SSI) benefits

SSI is a cash benefit paid by Social Security to people with limited income and resources who are blind, 65 or older, or have a disability. SSI benefits aren't the same as Social Security retirement benefits. You may be able to get both SSI benefits and Social Security benefits at the same time if your Social Security benefit is less than the SSI benefit amount, due to a limited work history, a history of low-wage work, or both. If you're eligible for SSI, you automatically qualify for Extra Help, and are usually eligible for Medicaid.

You can visit benefits.gov/ssa, and use the "Benefit Eligibility Screening Tool" to find out if you're eligible for SSI or other benefits. Call Social Security at 1-800-772-1213 or contact your local Social Security office for more information. TTY users can call 1-800-325-0778.

Note: People who live in Puerto Rico, the U.S. Virgin Islands, Guam, or American Samoa can't get SSI.

Programs for people who live in the U.S. territories

There are programs in Puerto Rico, the U.S. Virgin Islands, Guam, the Northern Mariana Islands, and American Samoa to help people with limited income and resources pay their Medicare costs. Programs vary in these areas. Call your Medicaid office (State Medical Assistance Office) to learn more. Visit Medicare.gov/contacts, or call 1-800-MEDICARE (1-800-633-4227) to get the phone number. TTY users can call 1-877-486-2048.

SECTION 8

Know your rights & protect yourself from fraud

What are my Medicare rights?

No matter how you get your Medicare, you have certain rights and protections. All people with Medicare have the right to:

- Be treated with dignity and respect at all times
- Be protected from discrimination
- Have personal and health information kept private
- Get information in a format and language they understand from Medicare, health care providers, Medicare plans, and Medicare contractors
- Have questions about Medicare answered
- Have access to doctors, other health care providers, specialists, and hospitals for medically necessary services
- Learn about their treatment choices in clear language that they can understand, and participate in treatment decisions
- Get Medicare-covered services in an emergency
- Get a decision about health care payment, coverage of services, or prescription drug coverage
- Request a review (appeal) of certain decisions about health care payment, coverage of services, or prescription drug coverage
- File complaints (sometimes called "grievances"), including complaints about the quality of their care

★ **Note:** Definitions of blue words are on pages 113–116.

What are my rights if my plan stops participating in Medicare?

Medicare health and prescription drug plans can decide not to participate in Medicare for the coming year. In these cases, your coverage under the plan will end after December 31. Your plan will send you a letter explaining your options. If this happens:

- You can choose another plan between October 15–December 7. Your coverage will begin January 1.
- **You'll also have a special right to join another** Medicare plan **until February 29, 2020.**
- You may have the right to buy certain Medigap policies within 63 days after your plan coverage ends.

What's an appeal?

An appeal is the action you can take if you disagree with a coverage or payment decision by Medicare or your Medicare plan. For example, you can appeal if Medicare or your plan denies:

- A request for a health care service, supply, item, or prescription drug that you think should be covered by Medicare.
- A request for payment of a health care service, supply, item, or prescription drug you already got.
- A request to change the amount you must pay for a health care service, supply, item, or prescription drug.

You can also appeal:

- If Medicare or your plan stops providing or paying for all or part of a health care service, supply, item, or prescription drug you think you still need.
- An at-risk determination made under a drug management program that limits access to coverage for frequently abused drugs, like opioids and benzodiazepines (see page 80).

If you decide to file an appeal, you can ask your doctor, supplier, or other health care provider for any information that may help your case. This will make your appeal stronger. Keep a copy of everything related to your appeal, including what you send to Medicare or your plan.

How do I file an appeal?

How you file an appeal depends on the type of Medicare coverage you have:

If you have Original Medicare

- Get the "Medicare Summary Notice" (MSN) that shows the item or service you're appealing. See page 52 for more information about MSNs.
- Circle the item(s) on the MSN you disagree with. Write an explanation of why you disagree with the decision. You can write on the MSN or on a separate piece of paper and attach it to the MSN.
- Include your name, phone number, and Medicare Number on the MSN. Keep a copy for your records.
- Send the MSN, or a copy, to the company that handles bills for Medicare (Medicare Administrative Contractor or MAC) listed on the MSN. You can include any other additional information you have about your appeal. Or, you can use CMS Form 20027. To view or print this form, visit CMS.gov/cmsforms/downloads/cms20027.pdf, or call 1-800-MEDICARE (1-800-633-4227) to have a copy mailed to you. TTY users can call 1-877-486-2048.
- You must file the appeal within 120 days of the date you get the MSN in the mail.
- You'll generally get a decision from the Medicare Administrative Contractor (MAC) within 60 days after they get your request. If Medicare will cover the item(s) or service(s), it will be listed on your next MSN.

If you have a Medicare Advantage or other Medicare health plan

The timeframe for filing an appeal may be different than Original Medicare. Learn more by looking at the materials your plan sends you, calling your plan, or visiting Medicare.gov/appeals.

In some cases, you can file a fast appeal. See materials from your plan and page 92.

If you have a Medicare Prescription Drug Plan

You have the right to do all of these (even before you buy a certain drug):

- Get a written explanation for drug coverage decisions (called a "coverage determination") from your Medicare drug plan. A coverage determination is the first decision your Medicare drug plan (not the pharmacy) makes about your benefits. This can be a decision about if your drug is covered, if you met the plan's requirements to cover the drug, or how much you pay for the drug. You'll also get a coverage determination decision if you ask your plan to make an exception to its rules to cover your drug.
- Ask for an exception if you or your prescriber (your doctor or other health care provider who's legally allowed to write prescriptions) believes you need a drug that isn't on your plan's formulary.
- Ask for an exception if you or your prescriber believes that a coverage rule (like prior authorization) should be waived.
- Ask for an exception if you think you should pay less for a higher tier drug because you or your prescriber believes you can't take any of the lower tier drugs for the same condition (or a lower tier drug isn't available).

How do I ask for a coverage determination or exception?

You or your prescriber must contact your plan to ask for a coverage determination or an exception. If your network pharmacy can't fill a prescription, the pharmacist will give you a notice that explains how to contact your Medicare drug plan so you can make your request. If the pharmacist doesn't give you this notice, ask for a copy.

If you're asking for prescription drug benefits you haven't gotten yet, you or your prescriber may make a standard request by phone or in writing. If you're asking to get paid back for prescription drugs you already bought, your plan can require you or your prescriber to make the standard request in writing.

You or your prescriber can call or write your plan for an expedited (fast) request. Your request will be expedited if you haven't gotten the prescription and your plan determines, or your prescriber tells your plan, that your life or health may be at risk by waiting.

Important! ▶ If you're requesting an exception, your prescriber must provide a statement explaining the medical reason why your plan should approve the exception.

What are my rights if I think my services are ending too soon?

If you're getting Medicare services from a hospital, skilled nursing facility, home health agency, comprehensive outpatient rehabilitation facility, or hospice, and you think your Medicare-covered services are ending too soon (or that you're being discharged too soon), you can ask for a fast appeal. Your provider will give you a notice before your services end that will tell you how to ask for a fast appeal. The notice might call it an "immediate appeal" or an "expedited appeal." You should read this notice carefully. If you don't get this notice, ask your provider for it. With a fast appeal, an independent reviewer will decide if your covered services should continue.

How can I get help filing an appeal?

You can appoint a representative to help you. Your representative can be a family member, friend, advocate, attorney, financial advisor, doctor or someone else who will act on your behalf. For more information, visit Medicare.gov/appeals. You can also get help filing an appeal from your State Health Insurance Assistance Program (SHIP). See pages 109–112 for the phone number.

What's an "Advance Beneficiary Notice of Noncoverage" (ABN)?

If you have Original Medicare, your doctor, other health care provider, or supplier may give you a notice called an "Advance Beneficiary Notice of Noncoverage" (ABN) if they think the care they'll provide isn't covered by Medicare. This notice says Medicare probably (or certainly) won't pay for some services in certain situations.

What happens if I get an ABN?
- You'll be asked to choose whether to get the items or services listed on the ABN.
- If you choose to get the items or services listed on the ABN, you're agreeing to pay if Medicare doesn't.
- You'll be asked to sign the ABN to say that you've read and understood it.
- Doctors, other health care providers, and suppliers don't have to (but still may) give you an ABN for services that Medicare never covers. See page 49.
- An ABN isn't an official denial of coverage by Medicare. If Medicare denies payment, you can still file an appeal. However, you'll have to pay for the items or services if Medicare decides that the items or services aren't covered (and no other insurer is responsible for payment).

Can I get an ABN for other reasons?
You may get a "Skilled Nursing Facility ABN" when the facility believes Medicare will no longer cover your stay or other items and services.

What if I didn't get an ABN?
If your provider was required to give you an ABN but didn't, in most cases, your provider must give you a refund for what you paid for the item or service.

Where can I get more information about appeals and ABNs?
- Visit Medicare.gov/appeals.
- Visit Medicare.gov/publications to view the booklet "Medicare Appeals."
- If you're in a Medicare plan, call your plan to find out if a service or item will be covered.

Your right to access your personal health information

By law, you or your legal representative generally has the right to view and/or get copies of your personal health information from health care providers who treat you, or by health plans that pay for your care, including Medicare. In most cases, you also have the right to have a provider or plan send copies of your information to a third party that you choose, like other providers who treat you, a family member, a researcher, or a mobile application (or "app") you use to manage your personal health information.

This includes:

- Claims and billing records
- Information related to your enrollment in health plans, including Medicare
- Medical and case management records (except psychotherapy notes)
- Any other records that contain information that doctors or health plans use to make decisions about you

You may have to fill out a health information "request" form, and pay a reasonable, cost-based fee for copies. Your providers or plans should tell you about the fee when you make the request. If they don't, you should ask. The fee can only be for the labor to make the copies, copying supplies, and postage (if needed). In most cases, you shouldn't be charged for viewing, searching, downloading, or sending your information through an electronic portal.

Generally, you can get your information on paper or electronically. If your providers or plans store your information electronically, they generally must give you electronic copies, if that's your preference.

You have the right to get your information in a timely manner, but it may take up to 30 days to fill the request.

For more information, visit hhs.gov/hipaa/for-individuals/guidance-materials-for-consumers/index.html.

If you need help getting and using your health records, the Office of the National Coordinator (ONC) in the U.S. Department of Health and Human Services (HHS) created "The Guide to Getting & Using Your Health Records." This guide can help you through the process of getting your health record and show you how to make sure your records are accurate and complete, so you can get the most out of your health care. Visit healthit.gov/how-to-get-your-health-record to view the guide.

How does Medicare use my personal information?

Medicare protects the privacy of your health information. The next 2 pages describe how your information may be used and given out, and explain how you can get this information.

Notice of Privacy Practices for Original Medicare

This notice describes how medical information about you may be used and disclosed and how you can get access to this information. Please review it carefully.

The law requires Medicare to protect the privacy of your personal medical information. It also requires us to give you this notice so you know how we may use and share ("disclose") the personal medical information we have about you.

We must provide your information to:
- You, to someone you name ("designate"), or someone who has the legal right to act for you (your personal representative)
- The Secretary of the Department of Health and Human Services, if necessary
- Anyone else that the law requires to have it

We have the right to use and provide your information to pay for your health care and to operate Medicare. For example:
- Medicare Administrative Contractors use your information to pay or deny your claims, collect your premiums, share your benefit payment with your other insurer(s), or prepare your "Medicare Summary Notice."
- We may use your information to provide you with customer services, resolve complaints you have, contact you about research studies, and make sure you get quality care.

We may use or share your information under these limited circumstances:
- To state and other federal agencies that have the legal right to get Medicare data (like to make sure Medicare is making proper payments and to help federal/state Medicaid programs)
- For public health activities (like reporting disease outbreaks)
- For government health care oversight activities (like investigating fraud and abuse)
- For judicial and administrative proceedings (like responding to a court order)
- For law enforcement purposes (like providing limited information to find a missing person)
- For research studies that meet all privacy law requirements (like research to prevent a disease or disability)
- To avoid a serious and imminent threat to health or safety
- To contact you about new or changed Medicare benefits
- To create a collection of information that no one can trace to you
- To practitioners and their contractors for care coordination and quality improvement purposes, like participation in Accountable Care Organizations (ACOs)

- We must have your written permission (an "authorization") to use or share your information for any purpose that isn't described in this notice. We don't sell or use and share your information to tell you about health products or services ("marketing"). You may take back ("revoke") your written permission at any time, unless we've already shared information because you gave us permission.

You have the right to:
- See and get a copy of the information we have about you.
- Have us change your information if you think it's wrong or incomplete, and we agree. If we disagree, you may have a statement of your disagreement added to your information.
- Get a list of people who get your information from us. The listing won't cover information that we gave to you, your personal representative, or law enforcement, or information that we used to pay for your care or for our operations.
- Ask us to communicate with you in a different manner or at a different place (for example, by sending materials to a P.O. Box instead of your home address).
- Ask us to limit how we use your information and how we give it out to pay claims and run Medicare. We may not be able to agree to your request.
- Get a letter that tells you about the likely risk to the privacy of your information ("breach notification").
- Get a separate paper copy of this notice.
- Speak to a Customer Service Representative about our privacy notice. Call 1-800-MEDICARE (1-800-633-4227). TTY users can call 1-877-486-2048.

If you believe your privacy rights have been violated, you may file a privacy complaint with:
- The Centers for Medicare & Medicaid Services (CMS). Visit Medicare.gov, or call 1-800-MEDICARE.
- The U.S. Department of Health and Human Services (HHS), Office for Civil Rights (OCR). Visit hhs.gov/hipaa/filing-a-complaint.

Filing a complaint won't affect your coverage under Medicare.

The law requires us to follow the terms in this notice. We have the right to change the way we use or share your information. If we make a change, we'll mail you a notice within 60 days of the change.

The Notice of Privacy Practices for Original Medicare became effective September 23, 2013.

How can I protect myself from identity theft?

Identity theft happens when someone uses your personal information without your consent to commit fraud or other crimes. Personal information includes things like your name and your Social Security, Medicare, credit card or bank account numbers, and your MyMedicare.gov user name and password. Guard your cards and protect your Medicare and Social Security Numbers. **Keep this information safe.**

Only give personal information, like your Medicare Number, to doctors, insurers or plans acting on your behalf, or trusted people in the community who work with Medicare like your State Health Insurance Assistance Program (SHIP). Don't share your Medicare Number or other personal information with anyone who contacts you by phone, email, or in person. Medicare, or someone representing Medicare, will only call you in limited situations:

- A Medicare health or drug plan can call you if you're already a member of the plan. The agent who helped you join can also call you.
- A customer service representative from 1-800-MEDICARE can call you if you've called and left a message, or a representative said that someone would call you back. If you suspect identity theft, or feel like you gave your personal information to someone you shouldn't have, call your local police department and the Federal Trade Commission's ID Theft Hotline at 1-877-438-4338. TTY users can call 1-866-653-4261. Visit ftc.gov/idtheft to learn more about identity theft.

How can I protect myself from fraud and medical identity theft?

Medicare fraud and medical identity theft can cost taxpayers billions of dollars each year. Medical identity theft is when someone steals or uses your personal information (like your name, Social Security Number, or Medicare Number) to submit fraudulent claims to Medicare and other health insurers without your permission. When you get health care services, record the dates on a calendar and save the receipts and statements you get from providers to check for mistakes. If you think you see an error or are billed for services you didn't get, take these steps to find out what was billed:

- Check your "Medicare Summary Notice" (MSN) if you have Original Medicare to see if the service was billed to Medicare. If you're in a Medicare health plan, check the statements you get from your plan.
- If you know the health care provider or supplier, call and ask for an itemized statement. They should give this to you within 30 days.
- Visit MyMedicare.gov to view your Medicare claims if you have Original Medicare. Your claims are generally available online within 24 hours after processing. You can also download your claims information by using Medicare's Blue Button. See page 103. You can also call 1-800-MEDICARE (1-800-633-4227). TTY users can call 1-877-486-2048.

If you've contacted the provider and you suspect that Medicare is being charged for a service or supply that you didn't get, or you don't know the provider on the claim, call 1-800-MEDICARE.

For more information, visit Medicare.gov, or contact your local Senior Medicare Patrol (SMP) Program. For more information about the SMP program, visit smpresource.org or call 1-877-808-2468.

You can also visit oig.hhs.gov or call the fraud hotline of the Department of Health and Human Services Office of the Inspector General at 1-800-HHS-TIPS (1-800-447-8477). TTY users can call 1-800-377-4950.

Plans must follow rules

Medicare plans and agents must follow certain rules when marketing their plans and getting your enrollment information. They can't ask you for credit card or banking information over the phone or via email, unless you're already a member of that plan. Medicare plans can't enroll you into a plan over the phone unless you call them and ask to enroll, or you've given them permission to contact you.

Important! **Call 1-800-MEDICARE to report any plans or agents that:**

- Ask for your personal information over the phone or email
- Call to enroll you in a plan
- Use false information to mislead you

You can also call the Medicare Drug Integrity Contractor (MEDIC) at 1-877-7SAFERX (1-877-772-3379). The MEDIC fights fraud, waste, and abuse in Medicare Advantage (Part C) and Medicare Prescription Drug (Part D) Programs.

Fighting fraud can pay

You may get a reward if you help us fight fraud and meet certain conditions. For more information, visit Medicare.gov, or call 1-800-MEDICARE (1-800-633-4227). TTY users can call 1-877-486-2048.

Investigating fraud takes time

Every tip counts. Medicare takes all reports of suspected fraud seriously. When you report fraud, you may not hear of an outcome right away. It takes time to investigate your report and build a case, but rest assured that your information is helping us protect Medicare.

What's the Medicare Beneficiary Ombudsman?

An "ombudsman" is a person who reviews questions, concerns, and challenges with how a program is administered, and helps to resolve them when possible.

There are several resources to get answers to your Medicare questions and get assistance with your Medicare, like Medicare.gov, 1-800-MEDICARE, and State Health Insurance Assistance Programs (SHIPs). The Medicare Beneficiary Ombudsman works closely with those resources and Medicare to help make sure information and assistance are available for you and works to improve your experience with Medicare.

Visit Medicare.gov for information on how the Medicare Beneficiary Ombudsman can help you.

CMS Accessible Communications

To help ensure people with disabilities have an equal opportunity to participate in our services, activities, programs, and other benefits, we provide communications in accessible formats. The Centers for Medicare & Medicaid Services (CMS) provides free auxiliary aids and services, including information in accessible formats like Braille, large print, data/audio files, relay services and TTY communications. If you request information in an accessible format from CMS, you won't be disadvantaged by any additional time necessary to provide it. This means you'll get extra time to take any action if there's a delay in fulfilling your request.

To request Medicare or Marketplace information in an accessible format you can:

1. **Call us:**
   For Medicare: 1-800-MEDICARE (1-800-633-4227)
   TTY: 1-877-486-2048

2. **Email us:** altformatrequest@cms.hhs.gov

3. **Send us a fax:** 1-844-530-3676

4. **Send us a letter:**
   Centers for Medicare & Medicaid Services
   Offices of Hearings and Inquiries (OHI)
   7500 Security Boulevard, Mail Stop S1-13-25
   Baltimore, MD 21244-1850
   Attn: Customer Accessibility Resource Staff

Your request should include your name, phone number, type of information you need (if known), and the mailing address where we should send the materials. We may contact you for additional information.

Note: If you're enrolled in a Medicare Advantage Plan or Medicare Prescription Drug Plan, contact your plan to request its information in an accessible format. For Medicaid, contact your State or local Medicaid office.

Nondiscrimination Notice

The Centers for Medicare & Medicaid Services (CMS) doesn't exclude, deny benefits to, or otherwise discriminate against any person on the basis of race, color, national origin, disability, sex, or age in admission to, participation in, or receipt of the services and benefits under any of its programs and activities, whether carried out by CMS directly or through a contractor or any other entity with which CMS arranges to carry out its programs and activities.

You can contact CMS in any of the ways included in this notice if you have any concerns about getting information in a format that you can use.

You may also file a complaint if you think you've been subjected to discrimination in a CMS program or activity, including experiencing issues with getting information in an accessible format from any Medicare Advantage Plan, Medicare Prescription Drug Plan, State or local Medicaid office, or Marketplace Qualified Health Plans. There are three ways to file a complaint with the U.S. Department of Health and Human Services, Office for Civil Rights:

1. **Online:**
   hhs.gov/civil-rights/filing-a-complaint/complaint-process/index.html.

2. **By phone:**
   Call 1-800-368-1019. TTY users can call 1-800-537-7697.

3. **In writing:** Send information about your complaint to:
   Office for Civil Rights
   U.S. Department of Health and Human Services
   200 Independence Avenue, SW
   Room 509F, HHH Building
   Washington, D.C. 20201

SECTION 9

Get more information

Where can I get personalized help?

1-800-MEDICARE (1-800-633-4227)

TTY users call 1-877-486-2048

Get information 24 hours a day, including weekends

- Speak clearly and follow the voice prompts to pick the category that best meets your needs.
- Have your Medicare card in front of you, and be ready to give your Medicare Number.
- When prompted for your Medicare Number, speak the numbers and letters clearly one at a time.
- If you need help in a language other than English or Spanish, or need to request a Medicare publication in an accessible format (like large print or Braille), let the customer service representative know.

Important! ▶ **Do you need someone to be able to call 1-800-MEDICARE on your behalf?**
You can fill out a "Medicare Authorization to Disclose Personal Health Information" form, so Medicare can give your personal health information to someone other than you. You can find the form by visiting Medicare.gov/medicareonlineforms or by calling 1-800-MEDICARE. You may want to do this now in case you become unable to do it later.

Did your household get more than one copy of "Medicare & You?"
If you want to get only one copy in the future, call 1-800-MEDICARE. If you want to stop getting paper copies in the mail, visit Medicare.gov/gopaperless.

⭐ **Note:** Definitions of blue words are on pages 113–116.

What are State Health Insurance Assistance Programs (SHIPs)?

SHIPs are state programs that get money from the federal government to give local health insurance counseling to people with Medicare at no cost to you. SHIPs aren't connected to any insurance company or health plan. SHIP staff and trained volunteers work hard to help you with these Medicare questions:

- Your Medicare rights.
- Billing problems.
- Complaints about your medical care or treatment.
- Plan comparison and enrollment.
- How Medicare works with other insurance.
- Finding help paying for health care costs.

See pages 109–112 for the phone number of your local SHIP. Contact a SHIP in your state to learn how to become a volunteer SHIP counselor.

Where can I find general Medicare information online?

Visit Medicare.gov

- Get information about the Medicare health and prescription drug plans in your area, including what they cost and what services they provide.
- Find Medicare-participating doctors or other health care providers and suppliers.
- See what Medicare covers, including preventive services (like screenings, shots or vaccines, and yearly "Wellness" visits).
- Get Medicare appeals information and forms.
- Get information about the quality of care provided by plans, nursing homes, hospitals, doctors, home health agencies, dialysis facilities, hospices, inpatient rehabilitation facilities, and long-term care hospitals.
- Look up helpful websites and phone numbers.

Where can I find personalized Medicare information online?

Register at MyMedicare.gov

- Manage your personal information (like medical conditions, allergies, and implanted devices).
- Sign up to get your "Medicare Summary Notices" (eMSNs) and this handbook electronically. You won't get printed copies if you choose to get them electronically.
- Manage your personal drug list and pharmacy information.
- Search for, add to, and manage a list of your favorite providers and access quality information about them.
- Select or change your primary doctor. Your primary doctor is the practitioner who you want responsible for coordinating your overall care, regardless of where you choose to get services. See page 105.
- Track Original Medicare claims and your Part B deductible status.
- Print an official copy of your Medicare card.

Still waiting for your new Medicare card?

1. Sign in to MyMedicare.gov to get your number or print your official card. Now that we've finished mailing new cards, your new number will appear in MyMedicare.gov.

2. Call 1-800-MEDICARE (1-800-633-4227). TTY users can call 1-877-486-2048. There may be something that needs to be corrected, like your mailing address.

You can only use your old card and Medicare Number to get health care services until December 31, 2019.

MyMedicare.gov's Blue Button®

MyMedicare.gov's Blue Button makes it easy for you to download your personal health information to a file. Having access to your information can help you make more informed decisions about your health care. Blue Button is safe, secure, reliable, and easy to use. By getting your information through Blue Button, you can:

• Download and save a file of your personal health information on your computer or other device, including your Part A, Part B, and Part D claims.

• Print or email the information to share with others after you've saved the file.

• Import your saved file into other computer-based personal health management tools.

Visit MyMedicare.gov to use Blue Button today.

Blue Button 2.0®

Medicare has released a new data service that makes it easy for you to share your Parts A, Part B, and Part D claim information with a growing list of authorized applications, services, and research programs. You authorize each application individually and you can return to MyMedicare.gov at anytime to change the way an application uses your information.

Once you authorize sharing of your information with an application (by using your MyMedicare.gov account information), you can use that application to view your past and current Medicare claims.

For Medicare Advantage Plans, only Part D information is available through this service. If you have a Medicare Advantage Plan, check with your plan to see if they offer a similar service to Blue Button 2.0.

Medicare keeps a list of authorized applications. Learn more by visiting Medicare.gov and searching for "Blue Button."

How do I compare the quality of health care providers?

Medicare collects information about the quality and safety of medical care and services given by most health care providers (and facilities).

Visit Medicare.gov/quality-care-finder and get a snapshot of the quality of care health care providers (and facilities) give their patients. Some feature a star rating system to help you compare quality measures that are important to you. Find out more about the quality of care by:

- Talking to your health care provider. Each health care provider should have someone you can talk to about quality.
- Asking your doctor or other health care provider what he or she thinks about the quality of care other providers give. You can also ask your doctor or other health care provider about the quality of care information you find on Medicare.gov.

Having access to quality and cost information up front helps you get a complete picture of your health care options. Later this year, Medicare.gov will have quality information in one easy-to-use place. You'll be able to compare quality ratings, cost information, and other details to help you get the best value for your health care.

How do I compare the quality of Medicare health and drug plans?

The Medicare Plan Finder at Medicare.gov/plan-compare features a star rating system for Medicare health and drug plans. The Overall Star Rating gives an overall rating of the plan's quality and performance for the types of services each plan offers.

For plans covering health services, this is an overall rating for the quality of many medical/health care services that fall into 5 categories and includes:

1. **Staying healthy—screening tests and vaccines:** Whether members got various screening tests, vaccines, and other check-ups to help them stay healthy.

2. **Managing chronic (long-term) conditions:** How often members with certain conditions got recommended tests and treatments to help manage their condition.

3. **Member experience with the health plan:** Member ratings of the plan.

4. **Member complaints and changes in the health plan's performance:** How often members had problems with the plan. Includes how much the plan's performance improved (if at all) over time.

5. **Health plan customer service:** How well the plan handles member calls and questions.

For plans that cover prescription drugs, this is an overall rating for the quality of prescription-related services that fall into 4 categories and includes:

1. **Drug plan customer service:** How well the plan handles member calls and questions.

2. **Member complaints and changes in the drug plan's performance:** How often members had problems with the plan. Includes how much the plan's performance improved (if at all) over time.

3. **Member experience with drug plan:** Member ratings of the plan.

4. **Drug safety and accuracy of drug pricing:** How accurate the plan's pricing information is and how often members with certain medical conditions are prescribed drugs in a way that's safer and clinically recommended for their condition.

For plans that cover both health services and prescription drugs, the overall rating for quality and performance covers all of the topics above.

You can compare the quality of health care providers and Medicare plan services nationwide by visiting Medicare.gov or by calling your State Health Insurance Assistance Program (SHIP). See pages 109–112 for the phone number.

What's Medicare doing to better coordinate my care?

Medicare continues to look for ways to better coordinate your care and to make sure that you get the best health care possible.

Here are examples of how your **health care providers** can better coordinate your care:

Electronic Health Records (EHRs)

EHRs are records that your doctor, other health care provider, medical office staff, or hospital keeps on a computer about your health care or treatments.

- EHRs can help lower the chances of medical errors, eliminate duplicate tests, and may improve your overall quality of care.
- Your doctor's EHR may be able to link to a hospital, lab, pharmacy, other doctors, or immunization information systems (registries), so the people who care for you can have a more complete picture of your health.

Electronic prescribing

This is an electronic way for your prescribers (your doctor or other health care provider who's legally allowed to write prescriptions) to send your prescriptions directly to your pharmacy. Electronic prescribing can save you money and time, and help keep you safe.

Accountable Care Organizations (ACOs)

An ACO is a group of doctors, hospitals, and/or other health care providers that work together to improve the quality and experience of care you get. ACOs help health care providers better coordinate your care and give you better quality care. Coordinated care saves time and costs by avoiding repeated tests and unneeded appointments. It may make it easier to spot potential problems before they become more serious—like drug interactions that can happen if one doctor isn't aware of what another has prescribed. Medicare evaluates how well each ACO meets these goals every year. Those ACOs that do a good job can earn a financial bonus. ACOs that earn a bonus may use the payment to invest more in your care or share a portion directly with your health care providers. Sometimes, ACOs may owe money to Medicare if their care increases costs.

An ACO can't limit your choice of health care providers. Your Medicare benefits aren't changing. You still have the right to visit any doctor, hospital, or other provider that accepts Medicare at any time, just like you do now. An ACO **isn't** a Medicare Advantage Plan, which is an "all in one" alternative to Original Medicare, offered by private companies approved by Medicare. An ACO **isn't** an HMO plan, or an insurance plan of any kind.

To help us coordinate your health care better, Medicare makes certain information about your care is available to ACOs working with your health care providers. Sharing your data helps make sure all the providers involved in your care have access to your health information when and where they need it. If you don't want Medicare to share your health care information in this manner, call 1-800-MEDICARE (1-800-633-4227). TTY users should call 1-877-486-2048. Even if you decline to share your health care information in this manner, Medicare will still need to use your information for some purposes, like assessing the financial and quality of care performance of the health care providers participating in ACOs.

If you have questions or concerns, you can talk about them during your office visit with your health care provider. For more information about ACOs, visit **Medicare.gov**, or call 1-800-MEDICARE.

Are there other ways to get Medicare information?

Publications

Visit Medicare.gov/publications to view, print, or download copies of publications on different Medicare topics. You can also call 1-800-MEDICARE (1-800-633-4227). TTY users can call 1-877-486-2048. Accessible formats are available at no cost. See page 99 for more information.

Social media

Stay up to date and connect with other people with Medicare by following us on Facebook (facebook.com/Medicare) and Twitter (twitter.com/MedicareGov).

Videos

Visit YouTube.com/cmshhsgov to see videos covering different health care topics.

Blogs

Visit Medicare.gov/blog for up-to-date information on important topics.

Other helpful contacts

Social Security

Find out if you're eligible for Part A and/or Part B and how to enroll, make changes to your Part A and/or Part B coverage, get a replacement Social Security card, report a change to your address or name, apply for Extra Help with Medicare prescription drug costs, ask questions about Part A and Part B premiums, and report a death.

1-800-772-1213, TTY: 1-800-325-0778
socialsecurity.gov

Benefits Coordination & Recovery Center (BCRC)

Contact the BCRC to report changes in your insurance information or to let Medicare know if you have other insurance.

1-855-798-2627, TTY: 1-855-797-2627

Beneficiary and Family Centered Care-Quality Improvement Organization (BFCC-QIO)

Contact your BFCC-QIO to ask questions or report complaints about the quality of care you got for a Medicare-covered service (and you aren't satisfied with the way your provider has responded to your concern). You can also contact your BFCC-QIO if you think Medicare coverage for your service is ending too soon (for example, if your hospital says that you must be discharged and you disagree). Visit Medicare.gov/contacts, or call 1-800-MEDICARE (1-800-633-4227) to get the phone number of your BFCC-QIO. TTY users can call 1-877-486-2048.

Department of Defense

Get information about TRICARE for Life (TFL) and the TRICARE Pharmacy Program.

TFL:
1-866-773-0404
TTY: 1-866-773-0405
tricare.mil/tfl
tricare4u.com

TRICARE Pharmacy Program:
1-877-363-1303
TTY: 1-877-540-6261
tricare.mil/pharmacy
express-scripts.com/tricare

Department of Veterans Affairs

Contact the VA if you're a veteran or have served in the U.S. military and you have questions about VA benefits.

1-800-827-1000, TTY: 1-800-829-4833
va.gov
vets.gov
eBenefits.va.gov

Office of Personnel Management

Get information about the Federal Employee Health Benefits (FEHB) Program for current and retired federal employees.

Retirees: 1-888-767-6738, TTY: 1-800-878-5707
opm.gov/healthcare-insurance

Active federal employees: Contact your Benefits Officer.
Visit apps.opm.gov/abo for a list of Benefits Officers.

Railroad Retirement Board (RRB)

If you get benefits from the RRB, call them to change your address or name, check eligibility, enroll in Medicare, replace your Medicare card, or report a death.

1-877-772-5772, TTY: 1-312-751-4701
rrb.gov

State Health Insurance Assistance Programs (SHIPs)

For free, personalized help with questions about appeals, buying other insurance, choosing a health plan, buying a Medigap policy, and Medicare rights and protections.

Alabama

State Health Insurance Assistance Program (SHIP)
1-800-243-5463

Alaska

Medicare Information Office
1-800-478-6065
TTY: 1-800-770-8973

Arizona

Arizona State Health Insurance Assistance Program (SHIP)
1-800-432-4040

Arkansas

Senior Health Insurance Information Program (SHIIP)
1-800-224-6330

California

California Health Insurance Counseling & Advocacy Program (HICAP)
1-800-434-0222

Colorado

State Health Insurance Assistance Program (SHIP)
1-888-696-7213

Connecticut

Connecticut's Program for Health Insurance Assistance, Outreach, Information & Referral, Counseling, Eligibility Screening (CHOICES)
1-800-994-9422

Delaware

Delaware Medicare Assistance Bureau
1-800-336-9500

Florida

Serving Health Insurance Needs of Elders (SHINE)
1-800-963-5337
TTY: 1-800-955-8770

Georgia

GeorgiaCares SHIP
1-866-552-4464 (option 4)

Guam

Guam Medicare Assistance Program (GUAM MAP)
1-671-735-7415

Hawaii

Hawaii SHIP
1-888-875-9229
TTY: 1-866-810-4379

Idaho

Senior Health Insurance Benefits
Advisors (SHIBA)
1-800-247-4422

Illinois

Senior Health Insurance Program
(SHIP)
1-800-252-8966
TTY: 1-888-206-1327

Indiana

State Health Insurance Assistance
Program (SHIP)
1-800-452-4800
TTY: 1-866-846-0139

Iowa

Senior Health Insurance
Information Program (SHIIP)
1-800-351-4664
TTY: 1-800-735-2942

Kansas

Senior Health Insurance
Counseling for Kansas (SHICK)
1-800-860-5260

Kentucky

State Health Insurance Assistance
Program (SHIP)
1-877-293-7447

Louisiana

Senior Health Insurance
Information Program (SHIIP)
1-800-259-5300

Maine

Maine State Health Insurance
Assistance Program (SHIP)
1-800-262-2232

Maryland

State Health Insurance Assistance
Program (SHIP)
1-800-243-3425

Massachusetts

Serving Health Insurance Needs
of Everyone (SHINE)
1-800-243-4636
TTY: 1-877-610-0241

Michigan

MMAP, Inc.
1-800-803-7174

Minnesota

Minnesota State Health
Insurance Assistance Program/
Senior LinkAge Line
1-800-333-2433

Mississippi

MS State Health Insurance
Assistance Program (SHIP)
844-822-4622

Missouri

CLAIM
1-800-390-3330

Montana

Montana State Health Insurance
Assistance Program (SHIP)
1-800-551-3191

Nebraska

Nebraska Senior Health
Insurance Information Program
(SHIIP)
1-800-234-7119

Nevada

State Health Insurance Assistance
Program (SHIP)
1-800-307-4444

New Hampshire

NH SHIP – ServiceLink
Resource Center
1-866-634-9412

New Jersey

State Health Insurance Assistance
Program (SHIP)
1-800-792-8820

New Mexico

New Mexico ADRC/SHIP
1-800-432-2080

New York

Health Insurance Information
Counseling and Assistance
Program (HIICAP)
1-800-701-0501

North Carolina

Seniors' Health Insurance
Information Program (SHIIP)
1-855-408-1212

North Dakota

State Health Insurance
Counseling (SHIC)
1-888-575-6611
TTY: 1-800-366-6888

Ohio

Ohio Senior Health Insurance
Information Program (OSHIIP)
1-800-686-1578

Oklahoma

Oklahoma Medicare Assistance
Program (MAP)
1-800-763-2828

Oregon

Senior Health Insurance Benefits
Assistance (SHIBA)
1-800-722-4134

Pennsylvania

APPRISE
1-800-783-7067

Puerto Rico

State Health Insurance Assistance
Program (SHIP)
1-877-725-4300
TTY: 1-878-919-7291

Rhode Island

Senior Health Insurance Program
(SHIP)
1-888-884-8721

South Carolina

Insurance Counseling Assistance
and Referrals for Elders (I-CARE)
1-800-868-9095

South Dakota

Senior Health Information &
Insurance Education (SHIINE)
1-800-536-8197

Tennessee

TN SHIP
1-877-801-0044
TTY: 1-800-848-0299

Texas

Health Information Counseling
and Advocacy Program (HICAP)
1-800-252-9240

Utah

Senior Health Insurance
Information Program (SHIP)
1-800-541-7735

Vermont

State Health Insurance Assistance
Program (SHIP)
1-800-642-5119

Virgin Islands

Virgin Islands State Health
Insurance Assistance Program
(VISHIP)
1-340-772-7368 St. Croix area;
1-340-714-4354 St. Thomas area

Virginia

Virginia Insurance Counseling
and Assistance Program (VICAP)
1-800-552-3402

Washington

Statewide Health Insurance
Benefits Advisors (SHIBA)
1-800-562-6900
TTY: 1-360-586-0241

Washington D.C.

Health Insurance Counseling
Project (HICP)
1-202-727-8370

West Virginia

West Virginia State Health
Insurance Assistance Program
(WV SHIP)
1-877-987-4463

Wisconsin

WI State Health Insurance
Assistance Program (SHIP)
1-800-242-1060

Wyoming

Wyoming State Health Insurance
Information Program (WSHIIP)
1-800-856-4398

SECTION 10

Definitions

Assignment
An agreement by your doctor, provider, or supplier to be paid directly by Medicare, to accept the payment amount Medicare approves for the service, and not to bill you for any more than the Medicare deductible and coinsurance.

Benefit period
The way that Original Medicare measures your use of hospital and skilled nursing facility (SNF) services. A benefit period begins the day you're admitted as an inpatient in a hospital or SNF. The benefit period ends when you haven't gotten any inpatient hospital care (or skilled care in a SNF) for 60 days in a row. If you go into a hospital or a SNF after one benefit period has ended, a new benefit period begins. You must pay the inpatient hospital deductible for each benefit period. There's no limit to the number of benefit periods.

Coinsurance
An amount you may be required to pay as your share of the cost for services after you pay any deductibles. Coinsurance is usually a percentage (for example, 20%).

Copayment
An amount you may be required to pay as your share of the cost for a medical service or supply, like a doctor's visit, hospital outpatient visit, or prescription drug. A copayment is usually a set amount, rather than a percentage. For example, you might pay $10 or $20 for a doctor's visit or prescription drug.

Creditable prescription drug coverage
Prescription drug coverage (for example, from an employer or union) that's expected to pay, on average, at least as much as Medicare's standard prescription drug coverage. People who have this kind of coverage when they become eligible for Medicare can generally keep that coverage without paying a penalty, if they decide to enroll in Medicare prescription drug coverage later.

Critical access hospital
A small facility that provides outpatient services, as well as inpatient services on a limited basis, to people in rural areas.

Custodial care
Non-skilled personal care, like help with activities of daily living like bathing, dressing, eating, getting in or out of a bed or chair, moving around, and using the bathroom. It may also include the kind of health-related care that most people do themselves, like using eye drops. In most cases, Medicare doesn't pay for custodial care.

Deductible
The amount you must pay for health care or prescriptions before Original Medicare, your prescription drug plan, or your other insurance begins to pay.

Demonstrations
Special projects, sometimes called "pilot programs" or "research studies," that test improvements in Medicare coverage, payment, and quality of care. They usually operate only for a limited time, for a specific group of people, and in specific areas.

Extra Help
A Medicare program to help people with limited income and resources pay Medicare prescription drug program costs, like premiums, deductibles, and coinsurance.

Formulary
A list of prescription drugs covered by a prescription drug plan or another insurance plan offering prescription drug benefits. Also called a drug list.

Inpatient rehabilitation facility
A hospital, or part of a hospital, that provides an intensive rehabilitation program to inpatients.

Lifetime reserve days
In Original Medicare, these are additional days that Medicare will pay for when you're in a hospital for more than 90 days. You have a total of 60 reserve days that can be used during your lifetime. For each lifetime reserve day, Medicare pays all covered costs except for a daily coinsurance.

Long-term care hospital
Acute care hospitals that provide treatment for patients who stay, on average, more than 25 days. Most patients are transferred from an intensive or critical care unit. Services provided include comprehensive rehabilitation, respiratory therapy, head trauma treatment, and pain management.

Medically necessary
Health care services or supplies needed to diagnose or treat an illness, injury, condition, disease, or its symptoms and that meet accepted standards of medicine.

Medicare Advantage Plan (Part C)
A type of Medicare health plan offered by a private company that contracts with Medicare. Medicare Advantage Plans provide all of your Part A and Part B benefits. Medicare Advantage Plans include:

- Health Maintenance Organizations
- Preferred Provider Organizations
- Private Fee-for-Service Plans
- Special Needs Plans
- Medicare Medical Savings Account Plans

If you're enrolled in a Medicare Advantage Plan:

- Most Medicare services are covered through the plan
- Medicare services aren't paid for by Original Medicare

Most Medicare Advantage Plans offer prescription drug coverage.

Medicare-approved amount
In Original Medicare, this is the amount a doctor or supplier that accepts assignment can be paid. It may be less than the actual amount a doctor or supplier charges. Medicare pays part of this amount and you're responsible for the difference.

Medicare health plan
Generally, a plan offered by a private company that contracts with Medicare to provide Part A and Part B benefits to people with Medicare who enroll in the plan. Medicare health plans include all Medicare Advantage Plans, Medicare Cost Plans, and Demonstration/Pilot Programs. Programs of All-inclusive Care for the Elderly (PACE) organizations are special types of Medicare health plans. PACE plans can be offered by public or private companies and provide Part D and other benefits in addition to Part A and Part B benefits.

Medicare plan
Any way other than Original Medicare that you can get your Medicare health or prescription drug coverage. This term includes all Medicare health plans and Medicare Prescription Drug Plans.

Premium
The periodic payment to Medicare, an insurance company, or a health care plan for health or prescription drug coverage.

Preventive services
Health care to prevent illness or detect illness at an early stage, when treatment is likely to work best (for example, preventive services include Pap tests, flu shots, and screening mammograms).

Primary care doctor

The doctor you see first for most health problems. He or she makes sure you get the care you need to keep you healthy. He or she also may talk with other doctors and health care providers about your care and refer you to them. In many Medicare Advantage Plans, you must see your primary care doctor before you see any other health care provider.

Referral

A written order from your primary care doctor for you to see a specialist or get certain medical services. In many Health Maintenance Organizations (HMOs), you need to get a referral before you can get medical care from anyone except your primary care doctor. If you don't get a referral first, the plan may not pay for the services.

Service area

A geographic area where a health insurance plan accepts members if it limits membership based on where people live. For plans that limit which doctors and hospitals you may use, it's also generally the area where you can get routine (non-emergency) services. The plan may disenroll you if you move out of the plan's service area.

Skilled nursing facility (SNF) care

Skilled nursing care and rehabilitation services provided on a daily basis, in a skilled nursing facility (SNF). Examples of SNF care include physical therapy or intravenous injections that can only be given by a registered nurse or doctor.

Notes

Help in other languages

If you, or someone you're helping, has questions about Medicare, you have the right to get help and information in your language at no cost. To talk to an interpreter, call 1-800-MEDICARE (1-800-633-4227).

العربية (Arabic) إن كان لديك أو لدى شخص تُساعده أسئلة بخصوص Medicare فإن من حقك الحصول على المساعدة و المعلومات بلغتك من دون أي تكلفة. للتحدث مع مترجم إتصل بالرقم MEDICARE-800-1 (4227-633-800-1).

հայերեն (Armenian) Եթե Դուք կամ Ձեր կողմից օգնություն ստացող անձը հարցեր ունի Medicare-ի մասին, ապա Դուք իրավունք ունեք անվճար օգնություն և տեղեկություններ ստանալու Ձեր նախընտրած լեզվով։ Թարգմանչի հետ խոսելու համար զանգահարեք 1-800-MEDICARE (1-800-633-4227) հեռախոսահամարով։

中文 (Chinese-Traditional) 如果您，或是您正在協助的個人，有關於聯邦醫療保險的問題，您有權免費以您的母語，獲得幫助和訊息。與翻譯員交談，請致電 1-800-MEDICARE (1-800-633-4227).

فارسی (Farsi) اگر شما، یا شخصی که به او کمک میرسانید سوالی در مورد اعلامیه مختصر مدیکردارید، حق این را دارید که کمک و اطلاعات به زبان خود به طور رایگان دریافت نمایید. برای مکالمه با مترجم با این شماره زیر تماس بگیریدMEDICARE-800-1 (4227-633-800-1).

Français (French) Si vous, ou quelqu'un que vous êtes en train d'aider, a des questions au sujet de l'assurance-maladie Medicare, vous avez le droit d'obtenir de l'aide et de l'information dans votre langue à aucun coût. Pour parler à un interprète, composez le 1-800-MEDICARE (1-800-633-4227)

Deutsch (German) Falls Sie oder jemand, dem Sie helfen, Fragen zu Medicare haben, haben Sie das Recht, kostenlose Hilfe und Informationen in Ihrer Sprache zu erhalten. Um mit einem Dolmetscher zu sprechen, rufen Sie bitte die Nummer 1-800-MEDICARE (1-800-633-4227) an.

Kreyòl (Haitian Creole) Si oumenm oswa yon moun w ap ede, gen kesyon konsènan Medicare, se dwa w pou jwenn èd ak enfòmasyon nan lang ou pale a, san pou pa peye pou sa. Pou w pale avèk yon entèprèt, rele nan 1-800-MEDICARE (1-800-633-4227).

Italiano (Italian) Se voi, o una persona che state aiutando, vogliate chiarimenti a riguardo del Medicare, avete il diritto di ottenere assistenza e informazioni nella vostra lingua a titolo gratuito. Per parlare con un interprete, chiamate il numero 1-800-MEDICARE (1-800-633-4227).

日本語 (Japanese) Medicare (メディケア) に関するご質問がある場合は、ご希望の言語で情報を取得し、サポートを受ける権利があります (無料)。通訳をご希望の方は、1-800-MEDICARE (1-800-633-4227) までお電話ください。

한국어(Korean) 만약 귀하나 귀하가 돕는 어느 분이 메디케어에 관해서 질문을 가지고 있다면 비용 부담이 없이 필요한 도움과 정보를 귀하의 언어로 얻을 수 있는 권리가 귀하에게 있습니다. 통역사와 말씀을 나누시려면 1-800-MEDICARE(1-800-633-4227)로 전화하십시오.

Polski (Polish) Jeżeli Państwo lub ktoś komu Państwo pomagają macie pytania dotyczące Medicare, mają Państwo prawo do uzyskania bezpłatnej pomocy i informacji w swoim języku. Aby rozmawiać z tłumaczem, prosimy dzwonić pod numer telefonu 1-800-MEDICARE (1-800-633-4227).

Português (Portuguese) Se você (ou alguém que você esteja ajudando) tiver dúvidas sobre a Medicare, você tem o direito de obter ajuda e informações em seu idioma, gratuitamente. Para falar com um intérprete, ligue para 1-800-MEDICARE (1-800-633-4227).

Русский (Russian) Если у вас или лица, которому вы помогаете, возникли вопросы по поводу программы Медикэр (Medicare), вы имеете право на бесплатную помощь и информацию на вашем языке. Чтобы воспользоваться услугами переводчика, позвоните по телефону 1-800-MEDICARE (1-800-633-4227).

Tagalog (Tagalog) Kung ikaw, o ang isang tinutulungan mo, ay may mga katanungan tungkol sa Medicare, ikaw ay may karapatan na makakuha ng tulong at impormasyon sa iyong lenguwahe ng walang gastos. Upang makipag-usap sa isang tagasalin ng wika, tumawag sa 1-800-MEDICARE (1-800-633-4227).

Tiếng Việt (Vietnamese) Nếu quý vị, hay người mà quý vị đang giúp đỡ, có câu hỏi về Medicare, quý vị sẽ có quyền được giúp và có thêm thông tin bằng ngôn ngữ của mình miễn phí. Để nói chuyện qua thông dịch viên, gọi số 1-800-MEDICARE (1-800-633-4227).

The information in "Medicare & You" describes the Medicare Program at the time it was printed. Changes may occur after printing. Visit Medicare.gov, or call 1-800-MEDICARE (1-800-633-4227) to get the most current information. TTY users can call 1-877-486-2048.

"Medicare & You" isn't a legal document. Official Medicare Program legal guidance is contained in the relevant statutes, regulations, and rulings.

Paid for by the Department of Health & Human Services.

U.S. DEPARTMENT OF HEALTH AND HUMAN SERVICES
Centers for Medicare & Medicaid Services
7500 Security Blvd.
Baltimore, MD 21244-1850

CMS Product No. 10050
Revised December 2019

PRSRT STD
POSTAGE & FEES
PAID CMS
PERMIT NO. G-845

National Medicare Handbook

Moving? Visit **socialsecurity.gov**, or call Social Security at 1-800-772-1213. TTY users can call 1-800-325-0778. If you get RRB benefits, contact the RRB at 1-877-772-5772. TTY users can call 1-312-751-4701.

¿Necesita usted una copia de este manual en Español?
Llame al 1-800-MEDICARE (1-800-633-4227). Los usuarios de TTY pueden llamar al 1-877-486-2048.

General comments about this handbook are welcome. Email us at **medicareandyou@cms.hhs.gov**. We can't respond to every comment, but we'll consider your feedback when writing future handbooks.

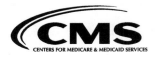